Drug Regimen
Compliance

Drug Regimen Compliance

Issues in Clinical Trials and Patient Management

Edited by

Jean-Michel Métry
AARDEX Ltd., Zug, Switzerland

and

Urs A. Meyer
University of Basel, Switzerland

JOHN WILEY & SONS

Chichester • New York • Weinheim • Brisbane • Singapore • Toronto

National   01243 779777   International   (+44) 1243 779777
e-mail (for orders and customer service enquiries): cs-book@wiley.co.uk
Visit our Home Page on http://www.wiley.co.uk or http://www.wiley.com

Commissioned in the UK on behalf of John Wiley & Sons, Ltd by Medi-Tech. Publications, Storrington, West Sussex RH20 4HH, UK

Co-publisher

Interpharm Press, Inc., 1358 Busch Parkway, Buffalo Grove, IL 60089, USA. International (+1) 708 459 8480

Other Wiley Editorial Offices

John Wiley & Sons, Inc., 605 Third Avenue, New York, NY 10158-0012, USA

WILEY-VCH Verlag GmbH, Pappelallee 3, D-69469 Weinheim, Germany

Jacaranda Wiley Ltd, 33 Park Road, Milton, Queensland 4064, Australia

John Wiley & Sons (Asia) Pte Ltd, 2 Clementi Loop #02-01, Jin Xing Distripark, Singapore 129809

John Wiley & Sons (Canada) Ltd, 22 Worcester Road, Rexdale, Ontario M9W 1L1, Canada

Library of Congress Cataloging-in-Publication Data

Drug regimen compliance : issues in clinical trial and patient
    management / edited by Jean-Michel Métry and Urs A. Meyer.
        p. cm.
    Includes bibliographical references and index.
    ISBN 0-471-97122-7 (cased)
    1. Patient compliance.   2. Drugs—Dosage.   3. Clinical trials.
    I. Métry, Jean-Michel.   II. Meyer, Urs A.
    [DNLM: 1. Patient Compliance.   2. Pharmaceutical Preparations–
    –administration & dosage.   3. Clinical Trials.   QV 771D7944 1998]
    R727.43.D78   1998
    615'.1—dc21
DNLM/DLC   98–28130
                                                              CIP

British Library Cataloguing in Publication Data

A catalogue record for this book is available from the British Library

ISBN 0-471-97122-7

Typeset in 10/12pt Baskerville from the author's disks by Dorwyn Ltd, Rowlands Castle, Hants
Printed and bound in Great Britain by Biddles Ltd, Guildford and King's Lynn
This book is printed on acid-free paper responsibly manufactured from sustainable forestry, in which at least two trees are planted for each one used for paper production.

Contents

Contributors

Ivo Abraham   *Center for Health Services and Nursing Research, School of Public Health, Catholic University of Leuven, Kapucijnenvoer 35/4, B-3000 Leuven, Belgium, Schools of Nursing and Medicine, University of Virginia, McLeod Hall, Charlottesville, VA 22903, USA*

Hans R. Brunner   *Division of Hypertension and Vascular Medicine, Lausanne University Hospital CHUV, CH-1011 Lausanne, Switzerland*

Michel Burnier   *Division of Hypertension and Vascular Medicine, Lausanne University Hospital CHUV, CH-1011 Lausanne, Switzerland*

Sabina De Geest   *Center for Health Services and Nursing Research, School of Public Health, Catholic University of Leuven, Kapucijnenvoer 35/4, B-3000 Leuven, Belgium*

Erik De Klerk   *University Hospital Maastricht, Department of Rheumatology, PO Box 5800, NL 6202 AZ Maastricht, Netherlands*

Jacqueline Dunbar-Jacob   *Center for Research in Chronic Disorders, School of Nursing, University of Pittsburgh, Victoria Building, Room 160, Pittsburgh, PA 15213, USA*

Claire-Lise Fallab Stubi   *Policlinique Médicale Universitaire and Division d'Hypertension et de Médecine Vasculaire, Rue César Roux 19, CH-1005 Lausanne, Switzerland*

Joerg Hasford   *IBE Department for Medical Informatics, Biometry and Epidemiology, Ludwig Maximilians University, Marchionstrasse 15, D-81377 Munich, Germany*

Guy Heynen   *Pfizer AG, Fluelastrasse 7, CH-8048 Zurich, Switzerland*

Jean-Marc Husson   *International Federation of the Associations of Pharmaceutical Physicians (IFAPP), 32 Avenue Duquesne, F-75007, Paris, France*

Dieter Magometschnigg   *Gesellschaft für Klinische Pharmakologie, Kinderspitalgasse 10, 15–17 A-1090 Wien, Switzerland*

Peter A. Meredith   *University Department of Medicine and Therapeutics, Gardiner Institute, Western Infirmary, Glasgow G11 6NT, UK*

Jean-Michel Métry   *AARDEX Ltd, Bundesplatz 10, Postfach 4149, CH-6304 Zug, Switzerland*

Urs A. Meyer   *Biozentrum der Universitat Basel, Abtlg. Pharmakologie, Klingelbergstrasse 70, CH-4056 Basel, Switzerland*

Carl Peck   *Center for Drug Development Science, Georgetown University Medical Center, 3900 Reservoir Rd NW, Washington DC 20007, USA*

Marie-Paule Schneider   *Policlinique Médicale Universitaire and Division d'Hypertension et de Médicine Vasculaire, Rue César Roux 19, CH-1005 Lausanne, Switzerland*

John Urquhart   *Pharmacoepidemiology Group, Department of Epidemiology, Maastricht University, NZ-6200 MD Maastricht, Netherlands*

Robert Vander Stichele   *Heymans Institute of Pharmacology, University of Gent, B-9000 Gent, Belgium*

Johan Vanhaecke   *Leuven Heart Transplant Program, University Hospital KU-Leuven, Herestraat 49, B-3000 Leuven, Belgium*

Wolfgang von Renteln-Kruse   *Reha-Zentrum Reuterstrasse, Geriatrische Klinik, Reuterstrasse 101, D-51467 Bergisch Gladbach, Germany*

Bernard Waeber   *Division of Hypertension and Vascular Medicine, Lausanne University Hospital CHUV, CH-1011 Lausanne, Switzerland*

Preface

Although patient compliance with drug regimens is hardly a new problem, renewed interest in this field during the past few years has been reflected by scientific meetings, new books, editorial comment, and many papers in peer-reviewed journals. Why the recent surge in interest, and why a new book?

In general, there is an overwhelming literature on compliance with drug regimens and it is difficult to obtain an overview. However, a recent bibliography of reviews[1], structured according to major compliance issues, indicated that there is a dearth of really new ideas, concepts, and perspectives due to a lack of adequate measurement methods in particular. It is by no means a new finding that insights into patient compliance depend on the method of measurement used[2]. Furthermore, it is the measurement technique which determines the definition of compliance. Another important point is that a knowledge of quantitative and qualitative features of non-compliance behaviour is a prerequisite for designing and testing appropriate measures for improving compliance. Most interestingly, a well proven measure of improving compliance with tuberculosis treatment, developed more than 30 years ago[3] (supervised therapy) is still of importance[4]. What, however, about new concepts for improving drug regimen compliance[5]?

Thus limited measurement methods hamper progress in compliance research, with regard to both descriptive and explanatory sides of the problem. A major point is that data from many previous studies revealed no relationship between compliance and the pharmacological effects of the drugs studied. In contrast, the results of many intervention studies were disappointing, only few showing any improvement in therapeutic outcome with compliance[6].

New techniques of compliance assessment, in particular those applying continuous microcomputer-based measurement, are giving us many valuable insights. Electronic compliance monitoring has enabled 'discovery' of new non-compliance behaviors, such as patient-initiated drug holidays[7], which obviously occur more often than anticipated. Interruptions to routine daily activities appear to be extremely critical to both the regularity and the consumption aspect of drug use[8,9]. Prescribed evening doses are more likely to be omitted or delayed than morning doses[10,11]. Furthermore, long-established assumptions about drug compliance have become questionable: for example, once-daily dosing may not necessarily be the best therapeutic option[9,12].

Most importantly, however, electronic compliance monitoring facilitated the generation of a much more meaningful definition of drug regimen compliance. Several aspects of patients' compliance behaviour can be quantified and analyzed in relation to the pharmacological properties of the drug studied[13].

This book is an overview of consequent developments, as well as challenges mainly derived from new insights into patients' compliance. It is also a 'perspective book', providing the basis for future steps in improving patient compliance and, by this, optimizing drug therapy and enhancing its safety.

Professor Ellen Weber, to whom this book is dedicated, died December 7 1992. She would have been very pleased by the recent advances in the research and understanding of drug compliance. In 1977, Professor Weber, previous head of the Department of Clinical Pharmacology at the Ruprecht-Karl University Heidelberg, initiated the very first compliance symposium in Germany[14]. In her studies she used different measurement methods[15–18]. Non-compliance is not restricted to ambulatory therapeutic settings, but also occurs among inpatients, as reported from studies including more than 1200 hospitalized patients. Ellen Weber's main interests concentrated on the safety of drug use[19,20]. She emphasized that compliance always should also be regarded in relation to safety issues[21]. Any evaluation of drug efficacy and safety is impossible without consideration of actual compliance. Therefore, Weber reiterated the demand for appropriate and reliable methods of compliance measurement in clinical trials as well as the need for consideration of patient compliance in medical practice[22,23].

Wolfgang von Renteln-Kruse
Reha-Zentrum Reuterstrasse, Geriatrische Klinik und Marien-Krankenhaus,
Bergisch Gladbach, Germany

REFERENCES

1. Van Campen C, Sluijs EM. *Bibliography patient compliance. A survey of reviews (1979–1989).* Den Haag: Netherlands Institute of Primary Health Care (NIVEL), CIP-Gegevens Koninklijke Bibliotheek, 1989.
2. Gordis L. Methodologic issues in the measurement of patient compliance. In: Sackett DL, Haynes RB, eds. *Compliance with therapeutic regimens.* Baltimore, London: The Johns Hopkins University Press, 1976, pp 51–66.
3. Fox W. Self-administration of medicaments: a review of published work and a study of the problem. *Bull Int Union Tuberc* 1962; **32:** 307–331.
4. Morse DI. Directly observed therapy for tuberculosis. Spend now or pay later. *BMJ* 1966; **312:** 719–720.
5. Haynes RB, McKibbon KA, Kanani R. Systematic review of randomised trials of interventions to assist patients to follow prescriptions for medications. *Lancet* 1996; **348:** 383–386.
6. Haynes RB, Wang E, Da Mota Gomes M. A critical review of interventions to improve compliance with prescribed medications. *Patient Educ Couns* 1987; **10:** 155–166.
7. Urquhart J, Chevalley C. Impact of unrecognized dosing errors on the cost and effectiveness of pharmaceuticals. *Drug Inform J* 1988; **22:** 363–378.

8. Vander Stichele RH, Thomson M, Verkoelen K, Droussin AM. Measuring patient compliance with electronic monitoring: lisinopril versus atenolol in essential hypertension. *Post Mark Surv* 1992; **6:** 77–90.

9. Kruse W, Rampmaier J, Ullrich G, Weber E. Patterns of drug compliance with medication to be taken once and twice daily assessed by continuous electronic monitoring in primary care. *Int J Clin Pharmacol Ther* 1994; **32:** 452–457.

10. Norell SE. Monitoring compliance with pilocarpine therapy. *Am J Ophthalmol* 1981; **92:** 727–731.

11. Kruse W, Nikolaus T, Rampmaier J, Weber E, Schlierf G. Actual versus prescribed timing of lovastatin doses assessed by electronic compliance monitoring. *Eur J Clin Pharmacol* 1993; **45:** 211–215.

12. Levy G. A pharmacokinetic perspective on medicament noncompliance. *Clin Pharmacol Ther* 1993; **54:** 242–244.

13. Urquhart J. The role of patient compliance in clinical pharmacokinetics. A review of recent research. *Clin Pharmacokinet* 1994; **27:** 202–215.

14. Weber E, Gundert-Remy U, Schrey A, Hrsg. Patienten Compliance Workshop am 14. Mai 1977 über Verbesserung der Arzt-Patienten-Beziehung in Frankfurt a.M. Baden-Baden, Köln, New York: Verlag Gerhard Witzrock, 1977.

15. Gundert-Remy U, Remy C, Weber E. Serum digoxin levels in patients of a general practice in Germany. *Eur J Clin Pharmacol* 1976; **10:** 97–100.

16. Gundert-Remy U, Möntmann U, Weber E. Studien zur Regelmäßigkeit der Einnahme der verordneten Medikamente bei stationären Patienten. *Inn Med* 1978; **5:** 78–83.

17. Fischer B, Lehrl U, Fischer U, Weber E. Drug compliance of progeriatric rehabilitation patients. Brief communication on a longitudinal investigation. *Akt Gerontol* 1983; **13:** 101–103.

18. Kruse W, Weber E. Dynamics of drug regimen compliance—its assessment by microprocessor-based monitoring. *Eur J Clin Pharmacol* 1990; **38:** 561–565.

19. Hollmann M, Weber E, eds. Drug utilization studies in hospitals. *A Satellite Symposium of the World Conference on Clinical Pharmacology and Therapeutics London, Wembley Conference Centre August 9, 1980.* Stuttgart, New York: FK Schattauer Verlag, 1981.

20. Weber E, Lawson DH, Hoigné R, eds. Risk factors for adverse drug reactions—epidemiological approaches. *Agents Actions* 1990; Suppl 29.

21. Weber E. Nicht Kontrolle, sondern mehr Sicherheit. *Münch Med Wschr* 1988; **130:** 56–57.

22. Weber E. Folgen inadäquater Therapie unter Berücksichtigung der Non-Compliance. *Arzneimitteltherapie* 1985; Suppl 1: 54–59.

23. Weber E. Introductory comment. First International Symposium on Compliance Monitoring, Heidelberg, June 6 1988.

1

Measuring Compliance in Clinical Trials and Ambulatory Care

Jean-Michel Métry

AARDEX Ltd., Zug, Switzerland

INTRODUCTION

Pharmaceuticals in ambulatory care are a leading interventional arm of modern medicine. The quality of their therapeutic and prophylactic use is thus a natural topic in considering the quality of health care.

The quality of pharmaceutical use involves such considerations as rational prescribing, identification of the optimal dosing regimen, avoidance of hazardous or effectiveness-compromising drug–drug or drug–food interactions and consideration of special patient characteristics such as liver or kidney disease or drug allergies that could either create hazard or nullify effectiveness. A closely related topic is the quality of the patient's execution of the prescribed pharmaceutical regimens. Obviously an untaken dose is an unabsorbed dose. Thus, non-compliance can be viewed as the ultimate absorption barrier[1].

Patient compliance with prescribed drug regimens is the focus of this book. It is a topic that occupies an ambiguous zone between patient and caregiver.

TERMINOLOGY—DIVERSITY REFLECTS AMBIGUITY AND AMBIVALENCE

The quality of the patient's use of prescribed drugs is variously termed 'patient compliance', 'patient adherence', 'observance' (in French), 'therapietrouw' (in Dutch, meaning 'faith with the therapy'), or 'concordance' (a recent suggestion)[2]. This proliferation of terms, each of which has its devotees

Drug Regimen Compliance: Issues in Clinical Trials and Patient Management.
Edited by J.-M. Métry and U.A. Meyer. © 1999 John Wiley & Sons Ltd.

and detractors, reflects the ambiguity of the topic and how it may impact on the roles of patient, doctor, pharmacist, nurse, and other caregivers.

Some see the topic as mainly a behavioral issue, focusing on the reasons why patients do not do as professionals believe they should; others see it as mainly a therapeutic issue, focusing on pharmacological consequences, treatment outcomes, and/or pharmacoeconomic impact in relation to different patterns of dosing. Some clinical researchers have held the view that patient non-compliance is a quality issue, akin to investigator non-compliance, but this view overlooks the fact that the patient is the experimental subject, not a member of the trial staff, so dose delays or omissions by experimental subjects are experimental results that must be reckoned with in the analysis.

A great deal of the ambiguity and divergence in viewpoint is attributable to confusion about the nature and extent of the problem, created by a long history of grossly inadequate methods for compiling accurate dosing histories of ambulatory patients. The dosing history is, by any reckoning, a logical starting point for a coherent discussion of discrepancies between the prescribed drug regimen and what the patient actually took, when. A natural consequence of poor methods is fuzzy definition of what is meant by 'non-compliance' or its various synonyms.

DEFINITIONS

A dosing history has the same parameters and physical dimensions as a drug regimen: how much is taken, and when. Because of this the regimen and the actual dosing history can be directly compared, to give rise to a precise definition of drug regimen compliance: the degree of correspondence between the actual dosing history and the prescribed regimen[3]. This comparison involves two time-series and is more involved than a simple comparison of two numbers, although the concept of 'Therapeutic Coverage' is a way of condensing a therapeutically salient aspect of the dosing history into a single number. This concept will be discussed later.

Until about a decade ago there was no way to capture reliable information on the timing of doses, and the topic of patient compliance as a field of either research or clinical practice was mired in methods that combined three bad properties: inaccuracy, imprecision, and bias. Inaccuracy arises from difficulties in recalling whether routine events were or were not performed. Imprecision arises from difficulties in specifying the times when doses were taken. Bias arises from the ease with which patients can hide evidence of omitted doses. A main focus of this chapter, and indeed the entire book, is how methodological advances have allowed the field to break free of these problems.

If adoption of the newer methods has been slower than might have been hoped, it is perhaps because the long-enmired grow fond of mud.

Non-compliance versus Discontinuation

A useful point of clarity is to draw a distinction between discontinuation and non-compliance. Discontinuation is, as its name implies, complete cessation of drug administration. Non-compliance implies continuation of dosing, albeit punctuated more or less often by lapses and occasionally by taking of extra doses. When a dosing lapse begins, only time can tell whether it will be permanent or a temporary 'drug holiday' that ends with resumption of at least an approximation of the regimen.

Early discontinuation of treatment is a common occurrence. Its consequences range from the trivial to the catastrophic, depending on drug, disease and its severity, and comorbidity. Early discontinuation is a major problem in ambulatory care: half or more of patients prescribed major types of chronic pharmacotherapy discontinue treatment within a year or two. It can have substantial economic consequences, for example when early discontinuation nullifies the values of a costly diagnostic workup and pre-discontinuation treatment. Sudden discontinuation of drug dosing may trigger hazardous rebound effects, although as a one-time event; patients with the holiday pattern of non-compliant dosing will be exposed to hazardous rebound effects and/or recurrent first-dose effects again and again.

An intriguing but unanswered question is whether the transition from punctual to erratic compliance is a precursor to discontinuation.

WHY METHODS ARE IMPORTANT

The history of the biomedical sciences is written in stepwise advances in methodology for measurement. Without adequate measurements progress is hardly possible but, when adequate methods do appear, knowledge expands rapidly. The topic of patient compliance is no different. It centers on compiling an accurate history of the patient's dosing—when the patient took which drug(s) and in what amounts—and the associated pharmacometric question of how the patient's dosing history projects itself into drug actions and therapeutic and economic outcomes.

As long as poor methods of monitoring remained in use, the topic of patient compliance remained scientifically dormant, and was the focus of only periodic expressions of opinion and repetition of unsubstantiated, ill-considered notions, unburdened by reliable data. Examples of such notions are:

- 'drug side-effects are the cause of non-compliance'
- 'once-daily dosing is the solution to the compliance problem'
- 'patient education is the solution to the compliance problem'
- 'patient empowerment is the solution to the compliance problem'

- 'multiple medications create compliance problems'
- 'patients with life-threatening diseases comply well'
- 'nothing can be done about poor compliance'
- 'my patients follow my instructions'.

None of these often-repeated assertions stand up to close scrutiny with sound methods, yet their continuing repetition reflects the ease with which the uncritical or uninformed offer opinions about compliance. Over the past decade, however, sound methods have built a body of solid evidence that renders obsolete the 'seems to me' school of commentary.

It is useful to understand the history of methods development, which this chapter undertakes to provide. There are basically three parts to the story: (1) interviews and other easily-censored methods, (2) chemical markers, (3) electronic monitoring. A fourth part shifts attention to the development of means of analyzing the data, which, because they are a time-series and not just a single number, require novel approaches.

EASILY CENSORED METHODS

The topic of patient compliance with prescribed drug regimens was initially popularized in the 1970s by a seminal book by edited by Louis Lasagna[4] and two books edited by David Sackett and Brian Haynes[5,6]. These early publications played an important role in creating awareness of the topic, but placed insufficient emphasis on the methodological problems that essentially stymied the field.

The methodological issues had already been brought into sharp focus a decade earlier by Alvan Feinstein and his colleagues, in the course of their work comparing alternatives for the prophylaxis of recurrent rheumatic fever[7-9]. In addition to its being a landmark study in the early development of clinical trials methodology, their study and analysis warrants revisiting, for the true pioneer of the field of patient compliance was not Sackett and Haynes, as many may think, but Feinstein. Unfortunately, Feinstein's work has been largely forgotten, mainly for three reasons: (1) it was done a long time ago; (2) rheumatic fever essentially disappeared within a few years of his work, a casualty of medical and public health progress; (3) his work was published earlier than the reach of most computerized search methods. Even so, it remains a landmark in the field.

Feinstein's Analysis

Feinstein and colleagues sought to determine the best regimen for anti-microbial prophylaxis of recurrent acute rheumatic fever. Depot penicillin, injected once monthly, was highly effective but the injection site became tender and painful for many days after the injection. In designing a trial to compare monthly depot and daily oral penicillin, they recognized that patient compliance would be a crucial issue, so they considered alternative means of assessing patients' dosing histories in their planned, 5-year trial of some 450 patients, all of whom had had at least one episode of acute rheumatic fever. The trial had three arms: monthly depot injections of penicillin; once daily oral penicillin; a control group (which, for ethical reasons, could not be a placebo) taking once-daily oral sulfadiazine, chosen on the grounds that it offered efficacy but lacked the bactericidal properties of penicillin[10].

Compliance with the monthly injection schedule for depot penicillin was driven to near-perfection by assiduous follow-up, which included pursuit and in-the-street injection of patients who skipped monthly clinic visits[10]. Injections were all administered by trial staff and duly recorded, providing an objective dosing history. Compliance with the oral regimen had to be measured by other means. Counts of returned dosage forms were considered but rejected, despite the superficial appeal of obtaining numerical data, because of the evident ease with which patients could censor evidence of delayed or omitted doses by simply discarding or hoarding untaken doses or by taking extra doses. Measurement of penicillin levels in blood or urine was rejected because the levels reflected drug intake during only a tiny fraction of the total treatment period. The method finally chosen was a series of interviews, one at each monthly visit, plus a semiannual review of the previous 6 months. A main focus of each interview was a consistency check: patients were continually asked to compare the past and prior months' compliance; similar comparisons were requested in the semiannual review. Another focus of each interview was to ascertain the sorts of cues or routines the patient used to insure timely dosing. The results supported a three-point scale: 'good', 'poor', 'doubtful'. In the final analysis, the 'doubtful' patients were combined with the 'poor', on the basis of the comparable clinical correlates in the two groups. About half the patients were in the 'good' category, the balance in the combined 'poor' and 'doubtful' category.

The results showed that, compared with poor compliers, good compliers with oral penicillin had a significantly lower incidence of both recurrent streptococcal infections and acute rheumatic fever. With sulfadiazine, good compliers had a much lower incidence of recurrent streptococcal infections than poor compliers, but the incidence of recurrent acute rheumatic fever was equally low in good and poor compliers alike—a difference that the authors did not comment upon, but which is probably the first reported instance of a 'forgiving' regimen[10].

Poor compliance with the depot injections was so infrequent that it was not possible to see whether good results could be obtained if some of the monthly injections were omitted[10]. The incidence of both streptococcal infections and acute rheumatic fever was lower in the recipients of depot penicillin than in good compliers with either oral penicillin or sulfadiazine. In subsequent studies, Feinstein and colleagues tried variations on the oral penicillin regimen in an effort to equal the results of the depot injections, but were never successful in doing so[10].

Additional Points

This trial showed several other noteworthy points.

1. Properly administered parenteral penicillin provided essentially complete prophylaxis against both types of disease in all patients randomized to receive the depot injections. It is noteworthy that about half of these patients bore all the behavioral and social factors that would have made them poor compliers had they been assigned to receive an oral medication. Nevertheless, the injected medicine worked effectively, despite whatever burdens there may be of having a 'non-compliant lifestyle'. In other trials, there are often circumstances in which poor results are not clearly attributable either to suboptimal dosing or to its behavioral correlates[11, 12], but here we see the medicine working in full force in virtually all patients assigned to receive it, despite roughly half of them having the behavioral correlates of poor compliance, as indicated by the compliance measurements in the patients assigned to receive the oral medications.

2. A second point is the surprisingly low incidence of acute rheumatic fever despite a high incidence of streptococcal infections in the poor compliers with sulfadiazine. This potentially important observation was ignored in the original reports of this work. Does sulfadiazine have some ability, apart from its antimicrobial action, to change the usual link between streptococcal infection and the induction of the autoimmune phenomena that give rise to acute rheumatic fever?

3. A plausible hypothesis for suboptimal prophylaxis in good compliers with oral penicillin is that continuity of penicillin action was occasionally compromised by a combination of oral bioavailability problems and/or occasional lapses in dosing that were undetected by the interview method.

4. Although not emphasized in the original work, good compliance was almost invariably associated with dosing being linked to some fixed, daily routine in the patient's life (Feinstein AR, personal communication). In other words, good compliance was virtually assured in patients who had robust routines, and who succeeded in linking the dosing regimen to one of those routines. This long-neglected finding can now be studied in a systematic manner, because we can now monitor actual dosing times. Knowledge of the time of day when dosing occurs (or does not occur) is crucial for understanding links, or lack thereof, between daily routines and dosing.

For various reasons, the approach taken by Feinstein and his colleagues was not followed by subsequent workers. Instead, two generations of clinical researchers have since relied on counts of returned dosage forms ('pill counts') as their measure of drug exposure in drug trials. The definitive evidence against 'pill counts' came in the late 1980s from studies with a low-dose phenobarbital marker.

CHEMICAL MARKER METHODS

In 1982, the US National Institutes of Health sponsored a workshop on chemical marker methods for assessment of drug regimen compliance by measurement of drug exposure in ambulatory patients. The conclusions to this conference[13] were apt in all but one respect, namely that the optimal marker should not 'accumulate' in the body. This conclusion reflected a concern that was acutely heightened that same year from the adverse experiences with the anti-inflammatory drug benoxaprofen, whose relatively long plasma half-life had, in some patients with outlying low clearance values, been a basis for a few extremely high concentrations of drug and associated toxicity. 'Accumulation' is a spectrum (for all drugs 'accumulate' to a certain extent in the body) inherent in the absorption–distribution–metabolism–excretion processes that govern pharmacokinetics.

The message from the workshop tended to point people toward the use of fast-turnover markers, which meant that the marker could reflect dosing only during only the 24–48 hours before plasma sampling. As was only discovered later, with electronic monitoring, this period happens to be the time when 'white-coat compliance' is most likely[14–16], i.e. the improvement in compliance around the time of a scheduled doctor visit. Thus, compliance during the previous 24–48 hours is upwardly biased relative to usually prevailing compliance.

Interpretation of Marker Data

The definitive work on marker interpretation was performed by Morgan Feely and his colleagues in Leeds[17–19]. Feely chose low-dose phenobarbital (phenobarbitone) because of its slow turnover, the remarkably low variance of its pharmacokinetic parameters, its long history of use, its relative safety, and the infrequency with which it is now used in clinical practice. Feely's papers[17–19] on the qualification of low-dose phenobarbital are models of what must be done with any other substance that one might contemplate using for a quantitative measure of drug exposure. The main issue in qualification is how to interpret marginally low concentrations of marker in plasma: are they reflective of low intake or of high clearance? Based on a careful analysis of the variance in the pharmacokinetic data on phenobarbital, Feely and his colleagues formulated a policy that in effect gave patients with borderline low marker concentrations the benefit of the doubt by calling them 'high-clearance outliers'.

Pharmacokinetic theory teaches that a single measurement of an agent's concentration in plasma basically reflects aggregate intake of agent during a period before the blood sampling equivalent to about three times the agent's plasma half-life[20]. In the case of phenobarbital this period corresponds to almost a week, minimizing the bias created by 'white-coat compliance'. Within that one-week 'time window', however, the method cannot indicate when doses were taken, but it surely documents the ingestion of marker-containing drug. The electronic monitors, in contrast, provide data on dose-timing, but cannot prove that doses were actually ingested.

The chief disadvantages of the marker methods are:

1. Repeated plasma samples are needed if compliance is to be documented over extended periods.
2. Special formulations are needed, with careful attention to minimizing the variance in marker content.
3. Special formulations must be validated by conventional bioavailability assessment of both drug and marker, and in terms of chemical stability over time.

These are not difficult issues, but they are costly ones, which should focus one's attention on the quality and utility of the data that can be provided by the marker, rather than by other methods.

Low-dose Digoxin Marker: The Helsinki Heart Study

The designers of the 4081-patient Helsinki Heart Study of the lipid-lowering agent gemfibrozil put much effort into a careful assessment of compliance. They included low-dose digoxin as a marker, along with a semiannual urinary measurement of drug in urine and returned tablet counts. Digoxin turns over about twice as fast as phenobarbital, and so the Helsinki data are probably somewhat inflated by white-coat compliance. When the Helsinki Heart Study was run, about one-third of patients were included in a special substudy in which the marker was used, along with counts of returned, unused dosage forms, and interviews. This work demonstrated the extent to which counts of returned dosage forms and interviews overestimate compliance[21].

A very important observation to come out of this work was the essentially identical distribution of compliance in patients assigned to receive the active drug (twice-daily gemfibrozil) and the placebo. This finding challenges the frequently made assertion that drug non-compliance is a consequence of side-effects.

The lipid-lowering effects of gemfibrozil varied in relation to drug intake, as assessed by the several methods used in the trial[22]. In Chapter 9 Urquhart analyzed the Helsinki Heart Study data in respect of the impact of variable compliance on the benefits and costs of treatment—less drug taken costs less to purchase, but less drug taken produces disproportionately smaller benefits; thus, the benefit/cost ratio deteriorates as compliance falls. These inter-relations are, however, specific to gemfibrozil. Obviously, a pharmaceutical whose daily dose is set far too high, as sometimes happens[22], could show a rise in the benefit/cost ratio as compliance falls until it reaches the dose optimum.

Another important result of the Helsinki Heart Study was that lipid lowering and coronary risk were independent of compliance with placebo[23]. This finding is important for several reasons. First, it shows that whatever 'lifestyle factors' may be coupled to the behavior that produces variable compliance, they have no discernible effect on the primary or secondary endpoints of this trial. Second, it reinforces the conclusion that the drug has dose-dependent efficacy. Third, examination of the relations between lipid lowering and compliance lead one to postulate that a higher dose might convey additional benefit.

Subsequent Work with Low-dose Markers

Feely and colleagues have published an array of studies using a low-dose phenobarbital marker to assess the prevalence and extent of suboptimal dosing and its clinical consequences in thyroid disease, rheumatoid arthritis, type II diabetes mellitus, coagulopathies, and other conditions[19]. Collectively, this work shows:

- the prevalence of poor and partial compliance
- the extent to which failed therapy is accounted for by poor compliance
- the extent to which clinical judgment underestimates poor compliance.

By inference, one may reasonably conclude that many patients are subjected to dose or drug escalations when the basic problem is not pharmacological non-response but non-compliance with previously prescribed medications.

These are the considerations that prompted development of electronic monitoring, which has gained wide acceptance as the 'gold standard' method for estimating drug exposure in ambulatory patients[24-27].

ELECTRONIC MONITORING

Electronic monitoring was pioneered at ALZA Corporation in the mid-1970s in the field of glaucoma management. Fred Glover, an engineer at ALZA, described an eyedrop container with integral time-stamping circuitry to record time and date when two events (cap removal and bottle inversion) coincide[28]. The Glover device was used by Kass and associates at Washington University to assess the compliance of glaucoma patients with topical pilocarpine eyedrops[15,29,30]. However, the Glover device, which was built just before major reductions in the size and power needs of electronic circuitry, was quite bulky in relation to conventional eyedrop dispensers, and so Kass's work was criticized on the grounds that the atypical device would change patient behavior. This criticism was refuted much later when much smaller devices, of typical eyedrop dispenser size, produced data entirely in keeping with Kass's first observations.

Several years later, Norell published work with another type of device, a conventional eyedrop container designed to sit in an electronically monitored cradle, which would record time and date when the container was removed from the cradle[31]. Norell's work, even though based on a doubly indirect method, captured the salient aspects of patient compliance in glaucoma— that underdosing through long intervals between doses was the predominant error, that there was a spectrum of errors (not simply a dichotomous all or none pattern of compliance/non-compliance), and that multiday lapses in dosing occurred in some patients from time to time. The data on compliance by glaucoma patients was essentially the same as compliance with a wide range of other chronically administered medications for hypertension, lipid lowering, inflammation, congestive heart failure, epilepsy, oral contraception, post-transplant immune suppression, HIV infection, and others[22]. Norell also grasped the fundamental point that the compliance data had to be interpreted in relation to the drug regimen: '... the aim of "improving" compliance is not to achieve perfect agreement between behavior and prescription, but to increase compliance only to the level where the outcome of treatment is improved. In practice, however, this level is often unknown...'[31].

Reconsidering that statement in light of what we know today, one might revise the wording thus: 'but to increase compliance only to the level where the sought-for outcome of treatment is achieved'. However, the wording change should not detract from the fundamental importance of the point.

In the mid-1980s Kass and colleagues published three papers based on studies in glaucoma patients with an eyedrop dispenser of usual size with fully integrated time-stamping microcircuitry[15,29,30]. The findings with this device hardly differed from those with the earlier bulky device or with Norell's results.

Taken collectively, the data from the three types of monitored eyedrop dispensers serve to negate the variety of criticisms that were voiced at the time each study was first presented, due to various imagined problems related to container size or whether the container was always replaced in the cradle, etc. One of the advantages of the eyedrop dispenser is that there is no way of removing doses ahead of time and carry them around in another type of container. It is, of course, possible that an occasional patient may alternate use of a monitored and a non-monitored dispenser but, like most of the postulated sources of artifact in electronic monitoring data, it is far from the path of least resistance, and thus unlikely.

Electronically Monitored Solid Dosage Form Containers

By 1985, the microelectronic revolution had reached the point that small computers were becoming ubiquitous, and size, costs, and power needs of microprocessors and other types of microcircuitry had fallen sufficiently to allow economic integration of time-stamping microcircuitry into normal-sized drug packages.

Urquhart has recently reviewed all aspects of the reliability of these devices, recounting the many technical problems that plagued early models: troublesome defects in plastic welds and solder joints, electrostatic discharge, and other problems that vexed those who sought to use these early devices, but which were typical problems of all microcircuitry-based products. These problems were eventually overcome, one by one. Today's electronic monitors have a failure rate of less than 1%.

Published Experience

There is now a literature of over 350 publications, including over 50 peer-reviewed original research papers, more than 30 symposium papers, 30 review articles, many book chapters, and over 125 abstracts of meeting posters or presentations. The only substantive criticism of the method in all this work has to do with conflicts that arise when a patient who prefers a dose organizer is asked to participate in a study involving the electronic monitor. Many of the patients who have incorporated one of the various dose-organizers into firm routines for insuring timely dosing will continue to use the organizer, loading it once weekly from the electronic monitor. Eventually monitoring will be integrated into one or more types of dose organizer; in the interim, researchers are advised to let patients use their familiar system, on the plausible assumption that their strong feelings reflect a strong commitment to, and achievement of, good compliance, and not try to force them into something they resist.

A recurring criticism of electronic monitoring is that it is an indirect method that cannot prove ingestion. This is true, but not apt, for it misses the fundamental point that the vast majority of patient errors are delays or omissions of doses—the scheduled time for dosing passes without the electronic signature of package entry. It could be that, in addition to the large numbers of such errors of omission detected in a large minority of patients, some undetected errors of omission are created when doses are removed from the package but not taken. That may be so in some instances, but it is no basis for changing the conclusions drawn from the electronic monitoring data. In contrast, what we have at present is wholesale reliance on tablet counts that grossly underestimate quantitatively and misspecify qualitatively the actuality of drug exposure in trials, lending false support to intent-to-treat averaging of drug responses that underestimates efficacy and hazard. In clinical practice we rely on clinical impression, which gives a similarly inflated view of drug exposure. The only reliable alternative to electronic monitoring is the low-dose, slow-turnover marker, which (as noted earlier) confirms ingestion but cannot show when doses were taken, and requires rather costly formulation and validation steps before it can be used.

Another point of criticism of electronic monitoring is the possibility that a patient might systematically open and close the container, and then discard the untaken drug. It is certainly possible to do so, but the patient must maintain this ruse daily for weeks or months in order to compile a false record of good compliance. An occasional patient may indeed do so, but it is an inherently unlikely form of malfeasance that, in the end, may have one patient in 50–100 misclassified as a 'drug non-responder'. In today's world, which relies substantially on clinical judgment in practice and returned tablet counts in trials, far more misclassified 'drug non-responders' succeed in presenting themselves as good compliers when in fact they are not. Several fraudulent investigators have learned how difficult falsification of evidence is, from their efforts to create false records of dose taking by manipulating the electronic monitors according to schedule[22].

DATA ANALYSIS

Time-series data have several important facets, which have been captured in a series of graphical displays that illuminate different aspects of a patient's dosing history. In the following examples (Figures 1.1–1.4), Figure (a) represents once-daily dosing and (b) three-times daily dosing.

Chronology Plot

The raw data can be displayed in a chronology plot, examples of which are shown in Figure 1.1. This view helps both patient and caregiver to focus on the nature of the patient's daily routines and how it may be possible to link dosing to some routine or other. The chronology plot also tells at a glance those patients who need help in achieving satisfactory correspondence between dosing history and prescribed regimen.

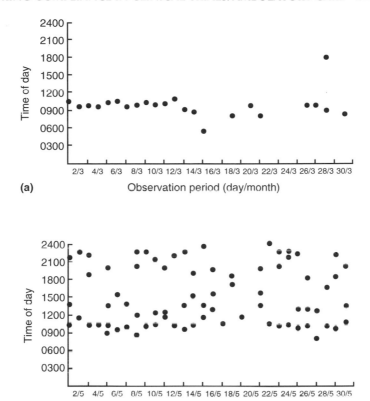

Figure 1.1 Chronology plots

For pharmacokinetic/pharmacodynamic simulation studies, the actual dosing history is the natural input to the model, as Rubio *et al.* were first to show[32]. As clinical trials simulation becomes more widespread, this use of the dosing chronology will inevitably grow, for one of the logical aims of trials simulation is to project the clinical and trial analytic consequences of the typical patterns of drug exposure.

Calendar Display

The calendar display suppresses data on the exact times of doses, giving instead a count of medication events within each 24-hour period. The result (Figure 1.2) looks like a conventional calendar, but shows the number of presumptively taken doses each day. As Norell was first to note, it is essential to end and begin the 24-hour 'day' at 3 a.m. instead of midnight, because this is for most patients a time of least activity. When the day ends and begins at a

	Mon	Tues	Wed	Thu	Fri	Sat	Sun
		1	1	1	1	1	1
7	1	1	1	1	1	1	1
14	1	1	0	0	1	0	1
21	1	0	0	0	0	1	1
28	2	0	1	1			

(a)

	Mon	Tues	Wed	Thu	Fri	Sat	Sun
							3
2	2	3	1	4	2	2	4
9	2	3	3	2	3	3	3
16	3	1	2	1	0	3	2
23	3	3	3	3	2	2	3
30	3						

(b)

FIGURE 1.2 Calendar display

busy time, then a minute or two's difference in dosing time on either side of the ending/beginning time may put one more or one less dosing event in the tally of the day's doses, creating the misimpression of highly variable compliance. These are called 'aliasing errors', and they are minimized when the 'day' changes at the time of least activity.

Frequency Histogram of Interdose Intervals

Yet another way to look at the data is to consider the frequency histogram of intervals between doses (Figure 1.3). The interval between doses has a special pharmacodynamic importance, because virtually all drugs stop working a certain period after the last-taken dose. Conversely, doses taken at too-short intervals will tend to push drug concentration in the plasma hazardously high.

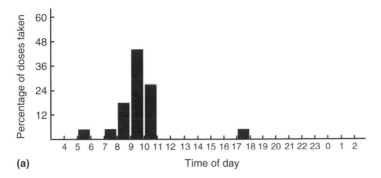

(a)

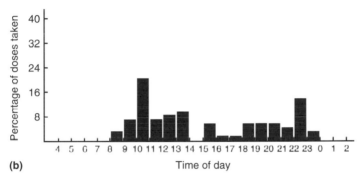

(b)

FIGURE 1.3 Frequency histogram of interdose intervals

Thus, both ends of the frequency histogram of interdose intervals convey useful information.

Therapeutic Coverage

An extension of this last point is the computation[33], of therapeutic coverage. To do so, one must know how long therapeutic drug action will persist after a dose, following a long enough period of dosing to create a 'steady state', typical of long-term pharmacotherapy. An illustrative example is provided by the combined estrogen–progestagen oral contraceptive, which, as interpreted by British regulators, has a 36-hour post-dose duration of action after which the risk of breakthrough ovulation begins to rise[34]. As long as each daily dose is taken at less than 36-hour intervals, sustained blockade of ovulation can be expected; this is the basis for the product's contraceptive action. When, however, the interdose interval exceeds 36 hours, then it may be said that therapeutic coverage has stopped, not to resume until shortly after the next pill is taken. The computation of therapeutic coverage proceeds by checking each interdose interval against the agent's post-dose duration of action, summing up those parts that exceed the agent's post-dose duration of action and expressing them as a percentage of treatment time. The complement of this, called therapeutic coverage, gives percentage of the treatment time during which the dosing history was sufficient to produce therapeutic drug action. It is also possible to create a frequency histogram of periods of inadequate drug action, on the expectation that many very short periods may have a different impact than a few quite long ones (Figure 1.4).

As new approaches in computer simulation of clinical trials develop, the construct of therapeutic coverage will probably attract widened attention, because it allows focusing on the periods of inadequate drug action and their clinical correlates.

Use of the therapeutic coverage concept serves to emphasize, however, how little we know about the post-dose duration of action of widely used drugs. One can only hope that appropriate studies to define this key parameter will become standard in new drug development. It took 35 years in the oral contraceptive field before such studies were performed, interpreted, and translated into drug labeling, which, in effect, tells patients how much compliance is enough, what the limits are, and what to do when one has gone past

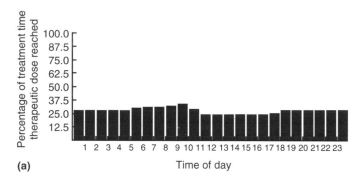

(a)

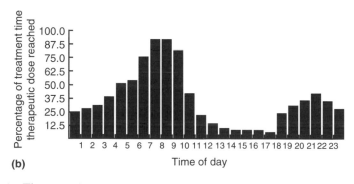

(b)

FIGURE 1.4   Therapeutic coverage

the limits[34]. A heartening development is that several post-dose duration of action studies have recently been carried out in the cardiovascular field[35–38], so we might soon begin to see labeling changes that convey information analogous to that provided to oral contraceptive users.

Electronic Tablet Counts

Electronic counting of medication events is superior to manual tablet counting, for the patient cannot tamper with the electronic record. The gross percentage of recorded doses can be examined relative to the prescribed number of doses to be taken within a specified interval. A rather more useful approach is to examine the percentage of treatment 'days' in which the prescribed number of doses were recorded as taken, because that percentage does not allow one to 'make up' for missing a dose one day by taking an extra dose some time later. Both days would be excluded from the tally of days on which the correct number of doses was taken.

Overview of Data Analysis

As Vrijens and Goetghebeur have pointed out[11], these time-series analyses pose novel problems for the analysis of clinical trials and the drug action correlates of variable dosing. The therapeutic coverage construct can, when there are adequate data to compute it, bring the whole story down to a single number, though one should take care not to oversimplify. Fortunately, the growing focus on clinical trials simulation should help to clarify how to make the most of this new capability.

Back to the Individual Patient

Recent work by de Klerk *et al.* teaches a useful way to search individual patient dosing histories for evidence that certain dosing patterns can trigger special responses[39]. They propose organizing individual patient data into a large spreadsheet in which each patient is a row and the columns depict, from left to right, patient identifiers and particular aspects of the dosing history (e.g. number of single days without dosing, number of two-consecutive-day periods without dosing, number of three-consecutive-day periods without dosing, number of days with one or more extra doses). Patients are rank-ordered by the parameter 'percentage of days with the correct number of doses taken'. Thus, patients near the top of the spreadsheet have few entries in columns to the right of the basic patient identifiers because they make few or no errors. In contrast, patients near the bottom of the spreadsheet have many entries in the columns to the right of the identifiers. The columns in the spreadsheet are made as detailed as seems necessary.

A next step is to make multiple copies of the spreadsheet and to devote each copy to the investigation of a particular clinical outcome, color coding patients with that outcome to see if particular outcomes cluster around certain dosing patterns. Outcomes of special interest are non-response, particular adverse events, and other unusual occurrences. A dosing correlate for any of these would logically serve as the basis for designing confirmatory studies, which may include pharmacodynamic studies in animals if ethical considerations preclude controlled studies in humans.

Some may dismiss this approach as a new form of 'data dredging', but this criticism ignores the fundamental property of all drugs, which is the dose- and time-dependence of their primary actions, and the time-dependence of counter-regulatory responses to those primary actions. An example is the complex time-course of the hazardous rebound effects that occur when dosing of beta-adrenergic blockers suddenly stops[40,41]. The occurrence of these rebound effects depends upon several conditions being met: (1) there has to have been sufficient previous drug exposure to induce receptor upregulation, without which there will be no rebound effects and (2) the interruption in dosing has to have been long enough to allow the blocking drug to disappear, after which (3) the patient enters a time-window of maximum risk, which is 10–14 days in length[40]. Thus the patient at greatest risk is probably one who occasionally punctuates otherwise fully compliant dosing with rather long drug holidays—probably at least 5 days—to allow time for receptor blockade to fade and then for episodes of sympathetic nervous system activation to occur and create the exaggerated catecholamine-driven responses that are the substrate for adverse coronary and other cardiovascular events[42].

Using this well documented example, and perhaps also some focused pharmacodynamic simulations, it is possible to design the spreadsheet's columns to facilitate discovery of dosing correlates of adverse events. This approach introduces the theme of dose pattern dependency to the investigation of infrequent adverse drug reactions.

CONCLUSION

The many chapters in this book present a variety of data from applications of electronic monitoring in many fields of therapeutics. What emerges from all this work is the view that, based on reliable measurements, electronic monitoring is the gold standard of measurement in this field and it is likely to expand rapidly. The ability to see daily and weekly patterns of dosing is a powerful tool previously unavailable for either trials analysis or patient management. A recent paper shows three typical patterns of dosing chronology over a period of about 6 weeks. The strictly punctual patient took each daily dose within minutes of the same time, every day. The slightly erratic patient delays the weekend dose by an hour or two. The completely erratic patient has little or no order in dose timing, and skips a number of doses. Such data can help patients and caregivers alike to find ways to establish daily routines for dosing, and thereby raise the standard of ambulatory pharmacotherapy so that many presently inadequately treated patients come under the umbrella of adequate treatment.

It is indeed an exciting prospect.

REFERENCES

1. Urquhart J. Non-compliance: the ultimate absorption barrier. In: *Novel Drug Delivery and its Therapeutic Applications*, eds LF Prescott and WS Nimmo. Chichester: John Wiley, 1989, pp 127–137.
2. Mullen PD. Overview, Royal Pharmaceutical Society Working Party on Concordance. *BMJ* 314: 691–2, 1997.
3. Urquhart J. Role of patient compliance in clinical pharmacokinetics: review of recent research. *Clin Pharmacokinet* 27: 202–15, 1994.
4. Lasagna L. ed. *Patient Compliance*. Mount Kisco, NY: Futura, 1976.
5. Sackett DL, Haynes RB, eds. *Compliance with Therapeutic Regimens*. Baltimore: Johns Hopkins University Press, 1976.
6. Haynes RB, Taylor DW, Sackett DL, eds. *Compliance in Health Care*. Baltimore: John Hopkins University Press, 1979.
7. Wood HF, Simpson R, Feinstein AR, Taranta A, Tursky E, Stollerman G. Rheumatic fever in children and adolescents: a long-term epidemiologic study of subsequent prophylaxis, streptococcal infections, and clinical sequelae. I. Description of the investigative techniques and of the population studied. *Ann Intern Med* 60 (Suppl 5). 6–17, 1964.
8. Gavrin JB, Tursky E, Albam B, Feinstein AR. Rheumatic fever in children and adolescents: a long-term epidemiologic study of subsequent prophylaxis, streptococcal infections, and clinical sequelae. II. Maintenance and preservation of the population. *Ann Intern Med* 60 (Suppl 5): 18–30, 1964.
9. Wood HF, Feinstein AR, Taranta A, Epstein JA, Simpson R. Rheumatic fever in children and adolescents: a long-term epidemiologic study of subsequent prophylaxis, streptococcal infections, and clinical sequelae. III. Comparative effectiveness of three prophylaxis regimens in preventing streptococcal infections and rheumatic recurrences. *Ann Intern Med* 60 (Suppl 5): 31–46, 1964.
10. Urquhart J. Ascertaining how much compliance is enough with outpatient antibiotic regimens. *Postgrad Med J* 68 (Suppl 3): S49–S59, 1993.
11. Vrijens B, Goetghebeur E. Comparing compliance patterns between randomized treatments. *Controlled Clin Trials* 18: 187–203, 1997.
12. Urquhart J, de Klerk E. Contending paradigms for the interpretation of data on patient compliance with therapeutic drug regimens. *Stat Med* 17: 251–67, 1998.
13. Insull W Jr. Workshop summary. *Controlled Clin Trials* 5: 451–8, 1984.
14. Kass MA, Gordon M, Meltzer DW. Can ophthalmologists correctly identify patients defaulting from pilocarpine therapy? *Am J Ophthalmol* 101: 524–30, 1986.
15. Cramer JA, Scheyer RD, Mattson RH. Compliance declines between clinic visits. *Arch Intern Med* 150: 1509–10, 1990.

16. Feinstein AR. On white-coat effects and the electronic monitoring of compliance. *Arch Intern Med* **150**: 1377–8, 1990.
17. Feely M, Cooke J, Price D, Singleton S, Mehta A, Bradford L, Calvert R. Low-dose phenobarbitone as an indicator of compliance with drug therapy. *Br J Clin Pharmacol* **24**: 77–83, 1987.
18. Pullar T, Kumar S, Tindall H, Feely M. Time to stop counting the tablets? *Clin Pharmacol Ther* **46**: 163–8, 1989.
19. Pullar T, Feely M. Problems of compliance with drug treatment: new solutions? *Pharm J* **245**: 213–5, 1990.
20. Benet LZ, Oie SS, Schwartz JB. Design and optimization of dosage regimens; pharmacokinetic data. In: *Goodman & Gilman's The Pharmacological Basis of Therapeutics*, Ninth Edition. Hardman JG, Limbird LE, Molinoff PB, Ruddon RW, Gilman AG, eds. New York: McGraw-Hill, 1996, p. 1729.
21. Maenpaa H, Manninen V, Heinonen OP. Compliance with medication in the Helsinki Heart Study. *Eur J Clin Pharmacol* **42**: 15–19, 1992.
22. Urquhart J. Comparative regulation of drug and of aircraft development: lessons for regulatory reform? *Clin Pharmacol Ther* **62**: 583–6, 1997.
23. Manninen V, Elo MO, Frick H, Haapa K, Feinonen OP, Heinsalmi P, Helo P, Huttunen JK, Kaitaniemi P, Koskinen P, Mäenpää H, Malkonen M, Manttari M, Norola S, Pasternack A, Pikkarainen J, Romo M, Sjoblom T, Nikkila EA. Lipid alterations and decline in the incidence of coronary heart disease in the Helsinki Heart Study. *JAMA* **260**: 641–51, 1988.
24. Vander Stichele R. Measurement of patient compliance and the interpretation of randomized clinical trials. *Eur J Clin Pharmacol* **41**: 27–35, 1991.
25. Kruse W. Patient compliance with drug treatment—new perspectives on an old problem. *Clin Invest* **70**:163–6, 1992.
26. Guerrero D, Rudd P, Bryant-Kosling C, Middleton BF. Antihypertensive medication-taking. Investigation of a simple regimen. *Am J Hypertens* **6**: 586–92, 1993.
27. Cramer JA. Microelectronic systems for monitoring and enhancing patient compliance with medication regimens. *Drugs* **49**: 321–7, 1995.
28. Glover F. US Patent 4,034,757, 1976.
29. Kass MA, Meltzer D, Gordon M, Cooper D, Goldberg J. Compliance with topical pilocarpine treatment. *Am J Ophthalmol* **101**: 515–23, 1986.
30. Kass MA, Gordon M, Morley RE, Meltzer DW, Goldberg JJ. Compliance with topical timolol treatment. *Am J Ophthalmol* **103**: 188–93, 1987.
31. Norell SE. Methods in assessing drug compliance. *Acta Med Scand Suppl* **683**: 35–40, 1984.
32. Rubio A, Cox C, Weintraub M. Prediction of diltiazem plasma concentration curves from limited measurements using compliance data. *Clin Pharmacokinet* **22**: 238–46, 1992.
33. Urquhart J. Therapeutic coverage: a parameter for analyzing the pharmacodynamic impact of partial patient compliance. *Program and Abstracts, Society for Clinical Trials/International Society for Clinical Biostatistics, Joint Meeting, Brussels, 1991,* p. 12.
34. Guillebaud J. Any questions. *BMJ* **307**: 617, 1993.
35. Johnson BF, Whelton A. A study design for comparing the effects of missing daily doses of antihypertensive drugs. *Am J Ther* **1**: 260–7, 1994.
36. Vaur L, Dutrey-Dupagne C, Boussac J *et al.* Differential effects of a missed dose of trandolapril and enalapril on blood pressure control in hypertensive patients. *J Cardiovasc Pharmacol* **26**: 127–31, 1995.

37. Leenen FHH, Fourney A, Notman G, Tanner J. Persistence of anti-hypertensive effect after 'missed doses' of calcium antagonist with long (amlodipine) vs short (diltiazem) elimination half-life. *Br J Clin Pharmacol* **41**: 83–8, 1996.
38. Hernandez-Hernandez R, Armas de Hernandez MJ, Armas-Padilla MC, Carvajal AR, Guerrero-Pajuelo J. The effects of missing a dose of enalapril versus amlodipine on ambulatory blood pressure. *Blood Press Monit* **1**: 1121–6, 1996.
39. de Klerk E, van der Linden S, van der Heijden D, Urquhart J. Facilitated analysis of data on drug regimen compliance. *Stat Med* **16**: 1653–64, 1997.
40. Rangno RE, Langlois S. Comparison of withdrawal phenomena after propranolol, metoprolol, and pindolol. *Am Heart J* **104**: 473–8, 1982.
41. Psaty BM, Koepsell TD, Wagner EH, LoGerfo JP, Inui TS. The relative risk of incident coronary heart disease associated with recently stopping the use of beta blockers. *JAMA* **263**:1653–7, 1990.
42. Houston MC, Hodge R. Beta-adrenergic blocker withdrawal syndromes in hypertension and other cardiovascular diseases. *Am Heart J* **116**: 515–23, 1988.

2

Design and Analysis of Clinical Trials of Compliance

Joerg Hasford
University of Munich, Germany

At some point, perhaps not in the far future, it will seem as wrong to run a clinical trial without compliance measurement as without randomization.

Bradley Efron[1]

INTRODUCTION

The history of compliance is as old as the traditional handing over of medical treatments. Even Hippocrates was aware that 'patients are often lying when they say they have regularly taken the prescribed medicine'[2]. From a behavioral point of view, compliance is defined as a patient's behavior in terms of taking medication, following prescribed diets, or executing medically recommended lifestyle changes[2]. In addition, compliance measures the extent to which a person's behavior coincides with medical or health advice. Thus, 'compliance' covers both a behavior and a measure. As the randomized trial is an experimental method of evaluating a drug's action, it seems wise to apply a pharmacokinetic and pharmacodynamic point of view: here, compliance is basically the quantitative indicator for a patient's drug exposure over time and its patient-dependent variation. Any physician-initiated deviations from the treatment regimens of the trial protocol are not covered by this definition, as there is usually a reason serious enough (e.g. lack of therapeutic action, adverse reactions) for deviation to occur. Such deviations do not fulfill the assumption of independence from prognosis, and, above all, compliance is a patient-centered concept.

As early as 1957, when the methodology of randomized trials was still in its childhood, Dixon *et al.* perceived and described the problems encountered with partial compliance in clinical trials[3]: 'Many chemotherapy trials based on unsupervised oral medication have probably been built on very unsure foundations. However carefully they were controlled statistically and scientifically,

Drug Regimen Compliance: Issues in Clinical Trials and Patient Management.
Edited by J.-M. Métry and U.A. Meyer. © 1999 John Wiley & Sons Ltd.

the results may have been vitiated by inadequate consumption of prescribed drugs.' Poor compliance may have been negligible or even beneficial for centuries, as long as almost no pharmacologically effective therapies were available. However, since the early days of the use of antibiotics, such as streptomycin, isoniazid, and penicillin, compliance has become an important issue of effective patient care[4].

Correct prescribing specifies the medicine, type of preparation, dosage, time, regularity, and method of application. More specific details may also be important (e.g. take before or after meals, avoid intake with dairy products). The physician may also ask the patient not to take certain other medicines: in clinical trials, such a prohibition is standard with regard to the respective control therapies.

Compliance assessments may be highly diverse. Patients can administer more or less than, or exactly as much, medicine as prescribed. Patients may take medicines erratically (sometimes taking more and sometimes less than prescribed). Finally, patients may neglect the recommended method of administration of the medicine or may take unauthorized medicines. Thus, compliance is a complex and heterogeneous construct.

IMPACT OF PARTIAL COMPLIANCE

Assuming the therapy under investigation being effective, partial compliance in clinical trials can lead to severe biases, which will—if neglected—result in incorrect judgments on efficacy, dose–response relationship, and safety:

- Partial compliance leads to an increased variability of the effect size and/ or to a diminished effect size (Figure 2.1). As a result, the power loss and the larger p-value lead to a false-negative decision. A possible cure is to increase the sample size, at least as long as the effect size is still clinically relevant. Above the excess financial burden (due to extra time and money) this may present an ethical problem: in trials with partial compliance the patient population must be larger—i.e. more patients are to be exposed to the inferior treatment than in trials with excellent compliance. Further possible scenarios are displayed in Figure 2.2.
- Partial compliance impairs the determination of the dose–response curve and of the lowest effective dose. To achieve a particular therapeutic effect, higher dosages are needed to compensate for partial compliance. As a result, the recommended dosage might later force compliant patients to overdose. Higher dosages, however, go along with a higher risk of adverse drug reactions. Additionally, higher recommended dosages mean higher treatment costs.
- Unrecognized partial compliance impairs the assessment of adverse events (Figure 2.3). Adverse events of the allergic or idiosyncratic type—type B reactions—are independent of compliance as long as the responsible drug

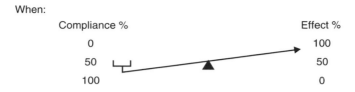

When:

Then: partial compliance
• increases variability of the outcome
• may bias size of outcome
• may thus bias the statistical test

FIGURE 2.1 Rationale for considering compliance to clinical trials

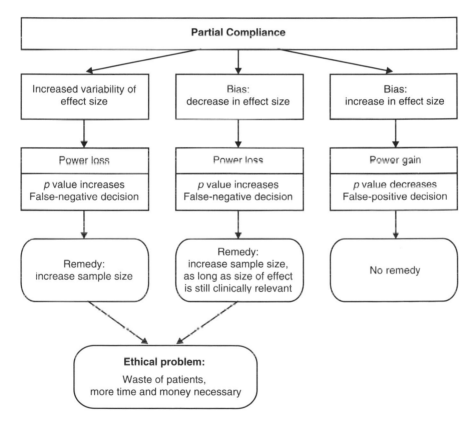

FIGURE 2.2 Impact of partial compliance on clinical trials

is administered at least once. However, the risk/benefit ratio is then negative as patients with a very low compliance suffer the risks of type B adverse reactions without the counterbalance of appropriate benefit.

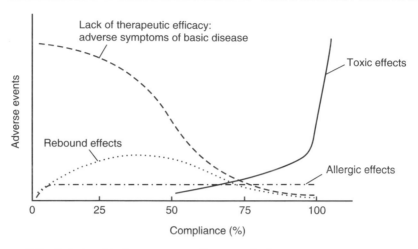

FIGURE 2.3 Relationship between compliance and adverse events

- Type A adverse events are dose-dependent by definition. Here, patients who administer more drug than prescribed, which is common for example in asthmatic patients, may suffer extra risks due to this 'hypercompliance', which may again not be counterbalanced by a corresponding higher benefit. Adverse events of the rebound-effect type present a particularly difficult problem. As there is usually a reverse temporal sequence, they occur only after treatment has stopped. Rebound adverse events are well known for beta-blockers and anticoagulants. Partial compliance is usually a repeated 'stop-and-go' therapy. Psaty *et al.* have shown that patients with poor compliance with beta-blocker treatment suffer from a considerably increased risk of fatal and non-fatal cardiovascular events[5].
- A further important source for wrong judgments are those adverse events which are symptoms or complications of the underlying disease, which has not been adequately treated due to partial compliance.
- Causality assessment of adverse events is questionable without compliance data, since prior drug exposure is a *conditio sine qua non* of an adverse drug reaction. Both the nominator and the denominator can be biased and the incidence cannot be truly determined. Most often the consequence will be an underestimation.
- Unrecognized and unaccounted partial compliance can thus severely distort the benefit/risk assessment.

USE AND METHOD EFFECTIVENESS

Sound empirical data verify that poor compliance goes along with a reduced therapeutic response in diseases such as hypertension[6], epilepsy[7], and infectious diseases[8].

Weis *et al.* have compared routine treatment and directly observed treatment of patients (DOT) with tuberculosis[8]. The DOT method implies that a health professional visits the patient every day, administers the medications and leaves only after having observed the patient take the medication. The DOT group can thus be regarded as a fully compliant group, whereas the group receiving routine care resembles in its compliance profile—varying from zero to perfect compliers—the typical groups of a randomized trial, which are analyzed following the intent-to-treat (ITT) strategy. Major outcome criteria were relapse rate and rate of acquired resistance. The relapse rate in the routine treatment group was about four times higher and the rate of acquired resistance seven times higher than in the DOT group (Table 2.1). The results of the routine treatment group ('use effectiveness') are identical to those that would have been received if only an ITT analysis had been performed. There is no doubt that the data from the DOT group show the importance of helping patients to become compliant. The results of the routine treatment group may lead to higher dosages and/or additional drug prescriptions.

Thus, it is essential to quantify the effect size of a particular treatment if it used correctly (i.e. by fully compliant people). This effect measure has been called 'method effectiveness'. Currently, as ITT analyses are the rule, only the use effectiveness data are provided, neglecting varying treatment exposures. Rational decision-making, however, calls for additional data about method effectiveness.

ITT ANALYSIS

The ITT analysis compares the outcomes of groups gained by random allocation irrespective of whether the treatments have been administered according to the study protocol. Not a single patient is to be excluded once he or she has been randomized. There are a couple of reasons—statistical and decision-theoretical—for ITT analysis. The ITT analysis protects the effects of randomization, it guards against statistically unbalanced groups and assures the validity of statistical tests. Above that, ITT analysis ideally provides the results seen in patients once the physician has decided to start a particular treatment.

TABLE 2.1 Rates of relapse and acquired resistance with the treatment of tuberculosis depending on compliance[8]

	Traditional therapy (partial compliance; $n = 407$)	Directly observed therapy (full compliance; $n = 581$)	p value
Relapse	20.9%	5.5%	0.001
Acquired resistance	10.3%	1.4%	0.001
	Use effectiveness	Method effectiveness	

These advantages do have their price, though. Populations and samples, respectively, may vary between studies with regard to disease, psychosocial and setting characteristics, resulting in varying compliance. Thus, the common ITT analysis of use effectiveness does not provide a valid and generalizable estimate of either the therapeutic effect size or of the risks. Two questions remain: what is the evidence of an ITT analysis, and to which populations can the results be transferred? Publications of clinical trials usually report very little information—if any—about demographic data, the amount of treatment actually administered, reinforcement of patients' compliance, or its success. These pieces of information are necessary to properly evaluate the outcome. The assessment of method effectiveness is essential and provides additional clinically useful information, as it standardizes one of the major impact factors—the size of treatment exposure.

Almost all papers on compliance data use in statistical analysis refer to the publication of the Coronary Drug Project (CDP) in 1980[9] as chief argument against using them.

The CDP analyzed survival rates of the groups receiving clofibrate and placebo in compliance-stratified subgroups (compliance below or above 80%). There was a clear positive compliance–effect relationship in the clofibrate group (5-year mortality 24.6% compared with 15%), with an almost identical placebo–compliance–effect relationship. In a long-term trial, however, such a positive placebo–compliance–effect relationship does not make sense. This result was considered to be an unavoidable artifact generated by subgroup analyses, and the authors' concluding statement represented the opinion still seen in major textbooks today: 'It is doubtful if any valid conclusions can be drawn from such analyses because there is no way of ascertaining precisely how or why the patients in the clofibrate and placebo groups have selected themselves or have become selected into the subgroups of good and poor adherers'[9].

A second, 'biometric' look at this publication, however, reveals major flaws, which invalidate these conclusions.

- There is no *a priori* hypothesis stating a correlation between compliance and treatment effect. This omission allows the results and conclusions to be regarded as a new hypothesis, which has to be examined subsequently before it can claim credibility.
- The methods used to 'assess' compliance do not meet any of the accepted quality criteria: validity, sensitivity, specificity, or representativeness. The highly unreliable pill count was used, mixed with the impressions of the physicians over a 5-year period, and averaged.
- For the statistical analysis, the quantitative compliance data are dichotomized in two arbitrary classes. No rationale for the cut-off point, 80%, is presented. Additionally, there is no evident reason why such a large sample (3760 patients) was divided into only two compliance strata.

- Many patients received effective non-trial medications such as nitrates, diuretics, and digoxin—i.e. clofibrate and placebo were served as adjunctive treatment. Compliance may be accounted equal for trial and non-trial drugs. This may explain the placebo compliance–effect relationship. This possibility has, however, not been discussed so far.
- Mortality risk after myocardial infarction is not constant but decreases over time. Thus, the impact of good compliance with effective drugs is much more profound the earlier the treatment is started. In this case it is clinically senseless to aggregate drug exposure data over the 5-year period into one number, irrespective of the time periods when drug exposure was more relevant with regard to the hazard rate.

It is obvious that the results of this publication cannot claim any empirical validity considering the inaccuracies of the methods chosen for compliance measurement.

From the clinical point of view, there is an urgent need to account for partial compliance when analyzing and interpreting clinical trials. However, the effects of proper randomization must be protected as far as possible, so that the bias induced by considering partial compliance is smaller than the bias resulting from the ITT analysis.

THE DECISION TREE

In the following section I will explain a set of criteria in the form of a decision tree[4], which can be used to decide whether the compliance measurement and the inclusion of compliance data into the statistical analysis make sense (Figure 2.4).

The basic idea of the criteria of the decision tree is to secure compliance data of sufficient quality and to check whether compliance must be regarded as a dependent variable or not. If there is evidence that in a particular trial compliance should be regarded as a dependent variable, then the compliance data cannot be used for the statistical analysis of the trial outcomes. In contrast to common expectations, there is little evidence that compliance is *per se* a dependent variable. Urquhart and De Klerk, for example, report that the compliance patterns are more or less the same across different diseases, treatments and patients[10]. If this is true patient compliance can be used as a baseline variable.

Trial Objectives

The first question of the decision tree asks for specification of the trial objectives: efficacy or effectiveness. In the context of clinical trials, efficacy (or

Decision Tree

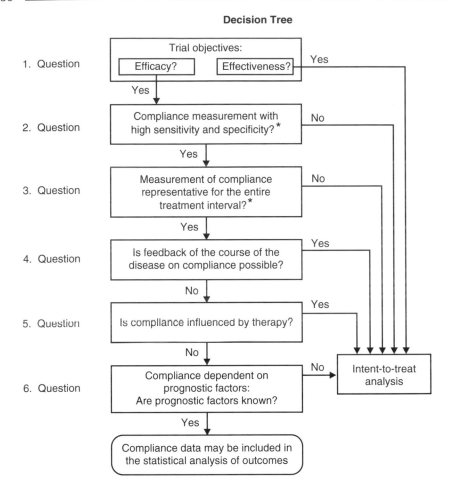

* Patients admitting to not having followed the prescribed therapy can be taken into account even if the measurement of compliance was otherwise unsatisfactory

FIGURE 2.4 A decision tree can be used to decide whether to include compliance data in statistical analysis

'explanatory approach') stands for the aim to find out whether and how a medicine works. Additionally, trial designers are supposed to look for ideal treatment conditions and to indicate the use of compliance data. 'Effectiveness' (or the 'pragmatic approach') looks for the beneficial and/or noxious effects of a particular treatment in routine clinical practice. One of the aims of such—usually late phase III or phase IV trials—is to find out whether a therapy will work despite partial compliance. This aim corresponds to the principle of the ITT analysis. Randomized trials with clinical endpoints that are usually performed after drug approval may, however, be considered as a mixture of the two, often demanding several different analyses[11].

Sensitivity and Specificity

The second question concerns 'sensitivity' and 'specificity' of compliance measurement. A more precise estimation of the treatment effects can only be achieved by *correct* measurements of the individual patient's compliance. Several studies demonstrated that all indirect methods of measurement, such as the common pill count, patient interview, impression of physician, and the presence or absence of a clinical response, provide only low to moderate sensitivity in the detection of non-compliance[4]. An important progress in compliance measurement even in a routine setting is represented by the electronic 'medication monitor'. The medication monitor is a pill box with an electronic device in its cover, which records each opening of the box by day, hour, and minute for up to 12–18 months. The medication monitor cannot prove that a medicine has actually been taken but if the pill box has been opened at regular intervals over a fairly long time period it seems reasonable to assume good compliance (whereas partial compliance can safely be supposed when the opening intervals deviate from the prescribed regimen and when the pill box contains more pills than it should). There will always be some patients who try to cheat the medication monitor, although it is hoped that these will be few[4].

Representativeness

This third criterion has largely been neglected[4]. Most treatments have to be administered repeatedly over time. Compliance measurement at a single (or a few) time points will not provide enough data to allow correct assessment of the patient's compliance at the different 'should be' time points of treatment administration. Thus, for a correct assessment of the compliance patterns of individual patients over time, compliance must be measured either at all 'should be' time points of treatment administration or at a representative sample of them. The latter will allow valid inferences regarding the population of 'should be' time points of treatment administration. Even direct methods of measurement at regular scheduled follow-up examinations will not generate the true pattern of compliance over time. Gordis *et al.* have compared physician visit compliance with compliance measured using direct methods at a random sample of treatment days[12]. Taking the random sample measurements as standard, the sensitivity of detecting non-compliance was 73%, and overall agreement existed for a mere 56% of the 103 patients. This study gives empirical evidence that compliance measurements using non-probability samples do not contribute to a precise statistical analysis because it would require correct compliance data. Including invalid compliance data into the statistical analysis can even be harmful since bias and wrong conclusions seem to be almost inevitable. *When compliance has not been, or will not be, assessed at probability samples or with the population of 'should be' time points of treatment administration, analyses should be restricted to the ITT approach.* From a biometric point of view this last criterion is extremely important: the validity of statistical analyses can in no case be better than the quality of the data themselves.

At present, only medication monitors can provide data that fulfill the requirements of this criterion. It seems practically unfeasible to assess compliance by drug or marker level monitoring for all 'should be' time points of a treatment intended to be administered repeatedly over time.

The impact of the following three criteria is not obligatory and respective problems can often be minimized by appropriate trial design.

Feedback

The eminent advantage of the randomized trial relative to its experimental character is that it provides a framework for reliable causal interpretation. One prerequisite is that the alleged cause precedes the effect. By introducing a variable into the statistical analysis of the outcome criteria as a stratifying factor or as a covariable that has been measured *after* the therapy has been administered, this prerequisite cannot safely be taken for granted[4]. Compliance will be considered as a dependent variable unless there is convincing evidence that it is not. Therefore, the fourth criterion demands careful checking of whether feedback on the course of disease on compliance was possible.

The empirical knowledge about feedback effects on compliance is limited and contradictory in the sense that both positive and negative feedback mechanisms have been reported[4]. A well known phenomenon is that an improving course of disease can have a negative feedback on compliance. In antibiotic trials, patients with disappearing infections often show poor compliance; thinking that antibiotics were harmful medicines, patients stopped taking them as soon as they felt better. Analyzing the relation between compliance and course of disease in a clinical trial when negative feedback is present produces the concept that the less medicine is taken, the more efficacious it is. The nonsense of this analysis is easily recognized but there are other possible effects of feedback mechanisms that are often difficult to detect as long as results are in accordance with present medical reasoning. When feedback mechanisms are probable the ITT analysis is indicated.

Compliance Influenced by Treatment

Criterion five also concerns causal interpretation. Compliance must enter the statistical analysis as a prognostic factor and not as an end in itself. This requires that compliance is an *independent* variable. Reasons for compliance being therapy-dependent may be a complex scheme of drug administration, safety devices of the drug package (e.g. childproof closures), or the patient's realization that they are taking placebo, to name just a few.

Compliance Influenced by Prognostic Profile

Attempts to integrate compliance data into the statistical analysis of outcome criteria aim to extract the true pharmacodynamic effects as precisely and in as unbiased a fashion as possible. Thus, a necessary condition is that compliance is not determined by prognostic factors: otherwise the observed change of the difference in effect size with better compliance cannot safely be explained only by the treatment—a different prognostic factor profile in the patients with better compliance is also probable. A prognostic factor is a variable measured *before* the start of treatment, which determines the course of disease. When no differences are found between treatment groups in the compliance distributions[8], it is usually reasonable to assume that the different compliance levels have not selected themselves based on different prognostic factor mixes between the treatment groups. It is important, however, to examine whether the different compliance levels represent heterogeneous prognostic factor mixes within a treatment group. The evidence gained by these analyses is as strong as the knowledge about prognostic factors. There are even diseases (such as vitamin or endocrine deficiencies) in which the main prognostic factor seems to be compliance with supplementary therapy itself.

The decision tree should not be used as an aid in deciding whether it is appropriate to integrate compliance data into the statistical analysis of the outcome criteria only after a trial has been completed[4]. From the biometric point of view, such decisions should be made early in the planning phase of a trial. The results of *a priori* planned analyses are obviously more convincing than of those performed *a posteriori*.

The aim of this set of criteria is to make rational decisions possible. Its use guarantees that the most important pitfalls will be considered.

IMPLICATIONS FOR THE STUDY DESIGN

As indicated by the decision tree, a study must be specifically designed to allow for the inclusion of compliance data in the statistical outcome analysis without introducing undue bias. First, it is absolutely essential to keep compliance as high as possible. There are many ways to promote compliance[13]. To start with, patients must be instructed exactly. The physician and his or her receptionist should explain the treatment regimen and ask the patient to repeat it in his or her own words. Handouts should support the spoken advice.

In long-term trials, these written instructions must be handed out at regular intervals. Patients need to be informed on how to proceed if they inadvertently miss out a dose. At the follow-up visit, the physician must question the patient about any difficulties in following the treatment regimen. The patient may need help to integrate the treatment into his or her daily routines. To improve compliance in clinical trials, much more can (and should be) done than is currently the rule. In the ideal situation—all patients being fully compliant—ITT analysis also provides an estimate of method effectiveness.

In some disease areas biofeedback tools can be used. Edmonds *et al.* have shown that self-measurement of blood pressure has a very positive impact on patient compliance[14]. The same may be true for self-measurement of peak flow by asthmatic patients.

Another design option is the run-in phase, in which compliance is examined for 4–8 weeks with either placebo or active treatment, before randomization. Only the good compliers are randomized. This pre-randomization compliance screen was used as early as 1967 in the Veteran's Administration Cooperative Study Group on Antihypertensive Agents, and later in the Physicians' Health Study and the SOLVD trial. The run-in phase seems to be especially indicated in long-term and intervention studies with expensive patient follow-up. There may, however, be problems with blinding, generalizability and the evaluation of the safety profile. For more details see Probstfield's review[15].

If compliance is expected to be far from perfect, sample size estimates should take this into consideration[16].

There is a variety of means of reducing or controlling the possible impact of feedback mechanisms on compliance. Many outcomes can be masked: for example, the patient does not feel high lipid levels, hypertension, lysis of gallstones, or conception unless the physician or a diagnostic test informs him or her. Another important tool for controlling possible feedback of the course of disease on compliance is to continuously measure outcome criteria, both beneficial and adverse, for example using automatic blood pressure and peak flow measurements and recording devices and electronic diaries. The electronic diary allows the patient to assess daily their physical function, pain or quality of life[17], and is simple to use. Thus, feedback mechanisms, if there are any, can be properly assessed and used for the joint interpretation of compliance and outcome data.

As compliance should be independent of therapy in a technical sense (packaging, dosages per day, galenic formulation etc.), technical details should be kept as similar as possible across treatment and control groups, unless the use of different modes of presentation is one of the research questions.

Finally, one should try to find out the reasons for partial compliance, either by interview or self-administered questionnaires. This provides important information on how to use and interpret compliance data in the context of outcome analysis.

STATISTICAL ANALYSIS

The statistical analysis should be transparent, and as simple as possible without oversimplifying. Close cooperation between a clinician or clinical pharmacologist and a biostatistician will most often be needed as the statistical procedure has to be tailored for the particular study. Thus, only some general principles can be given here.

The major aims of using compliance data as an independent variable in the statistical analysis are:

- to adjust the statistical tests for the impact of partial compliance;
- to estimate the treatment effect size under the assumption of 100% compliance;
- to identify the compliance that is necessary to achieve therapeutic benefit;
- to specify the dose–response relationship
- to improve the assessment of therapy-related risks (e.g. causality, incidence).

Indexing Compliance Data

The first problem to be solved is how to aggregate the repeated measurements of compliance[10,18]. Compliance can be calculated as the number of days at which all prescribed doses have been administered divided by the number of days of the treatment period, or as the number of doses actually administered divided by the number of all doses prescribed. If reliable data for the duration of drug action are available the time intervals between drug administrations can be used to calculate an index called 'timing compliance'. One should also consider the pattern of compliance and the possibly different impact of compliance on the course of disease over time. From a medical point of view, it can be highly relevant whether a patient is compliant during the first phase of therapy and non-compliant in the second (or vice versa), or whether the patient omits every second dose. The resulting course of disease (measured as therapeutic efficacy) may be different, although the compliance index may be the same for all different compliance patterns. It should also be remembered that the time window of maximum possible treatment efficacy must not stretch over the whole treatment period (e.g. the risk of reinfarction is higher during the first 6 months after myocardial infarction than afterwards, thus compliance with therapy during the first 6 months is more important than later). The common practice of averaging compliance results over the whole treatment period may lead to considerable bias[4].

A solution to this might be hierarchical ranking of the different compliance patterns with respect to the *a priori* knowledge about the pharmacodynamics and pharmacokinetics of the particular medicines and about the impact of treatment, which may vary during the course of the disease. Unless there are reliable pharmacological data dichotomizations of compliance, such as the common ≥80% and <80% cutoff points, must be avoided.

Analysis of Compliance Distributions and Interactions

The next step is to compare the compliance distributions across the trial groups, prognostic subgroups and over time in order to check whether there is an interaction between treatment or prognostic profile and compliance. If a statistical test is used and a significant difference shown it is important to determine whether the difference in the compliance distributions has real relevance, especially if the sample sizes are large. The disadvantage of the statistical test is that when the null hypothesis is retained one must not conclude that it is true. Thus, it might be advisable to apply descriptively the procedures common in assessing bioequivalence. If there is a relevant interaction to be seen, further analyses might provide weak evidence only, as it will be difficult to separate and measure the respective impact of these covariates. Thus, the ITT analysis is appropriate.

The effect size in the strata of very low or zero compliance should also be checked. Ideally, there should be no differences across the groups, as there was no or only minor treatment exposure. Significant differences are a serious hint of an interaction between prognostic profile and compliance. Unless the prognostic factors are very well known, so that adequate statistical adjustment techniques can be used, the ITT analysis should be followed.

EXAMINING THE COMPLIANCE–EFFECT-SIZE RELATIONSHIP

Effect size should be displayed for varying degrees of compliance. The stronger the correlation or the steeper the slope, the more promising will be the analysis. If no, or only a minor, relationship can be seen further analyses will usually not make sense. There are a couple of reasons for such a no-relation observation: the treatment might not be efficacious, the dosage chosen or the mode of action might make partial compliance irrelevant (forgiving drugs[10]). If the attempts to reinforce compliance were successful, variability of compliance in the trial samples might be too small to show any relationship.

When the effect size for almost perfect and perfect compliance displays a plateau, dosage reduction might be possible; otherwise a higher dosage might produce a greater effect size.

These descriptive techniques may be simple but they are essential to disclose hidden information in the outcome data, and most clinicians will understand them.

Adjusting the Statistical Test for Partial Compliance

For the adjustment of statistical tests there is a large array of standard techniques (e.g. Mantel–Haenszel test, logistic regression, analysis of covariance, Cox model) for using covariates; these depend mainly on the type and distribution of the covariate and the outcome variable. It is absolutely essential, however, that not a single patient is excluded from these analyses because they are a poor or partial complier. In addition, to achieve acceptance of the result of these analyses, it is vital to ensure transparency of the whole statistical procedure and to use, whenever possible, familiar and accepted statistical techniques.

In recent years sophisticated statistical models requiring advanced computing capabilities, have been proposed[19]. Efron and Feldmann have reanalyzed the Lipid Research Clinics Coronary Primary Prevention Trial (LRC-CPPT) data with the aim of extracting an unbiased compliance–response relationship[20]. Rubin's key idea was to obtain a p value using a posterior predictive check distribution, which includes a model for non-compliance behavior, although only under the sharp null hypothesis of 'no effect of assignment or receipt of treatment on outcome'[21]. Goetghebeur has used and compared several techniques for a variety of trials[22,23], some with compliance data of questionable quality and focusing on physician initiated changes of treatment[24], a topic not covered by the definition of patient compliance given in this chapter. With regard to equivalence trials, Robins presents various structural models assuming that the patient's decision whether or not to continue to comply with the randomly allocated treatment is random conditional on the history of measured prerandomization and time-dependent post-randomization prognostic factors[25].

CONCLUSIONS

The US Food and Drug Administration has approved a display in the patient information leaflet (PIL) of the relationship between compliance with cholestyramine, coronary risk reduction and reduction in total cholesterol level derived from LRC-CPPT data[26] (Figure 2.5). Perfectly compliant patients might expect a reduction in coronary risk of about 40%, whereas averagely compliant patients yield a risk reduction of only approximately 20%. This is an important piece of information which the patient has a right to know. (There is an interesting asymmetry: the frequency and severity of adverse drug reactions is often quantified in the PIL, whereas the beneficial effects are not!)

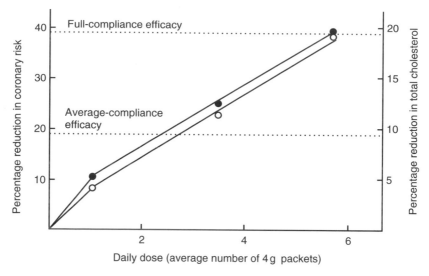

FIGURE 2.5 Percentage reduction in coronary risk (●) and total cholesterol level (○) related to dose of cholestyramine

In theory, there may be countless reasons for not using compliance data but there are very few, if any, valid empirical data for this negligence. Nowadays, many drugs really work and drug exposure will become *the* major covariable, irrespective of most patient characteristics. Oral contraceptives, for example, do completely protect (if properly administered) all women taking them, irrespective of their beliefs, habits, attitudes, risk profile and other characteristics.

I have not gone into details with regard to adverse events and adverse drug reactions: real-time compliance measurements help a more valid single case causality assessments. In addition, the nominator and the denominator can be adjusted according to the extent of drug exposure.

In conclusion, biometricians are asked to provide adequate trial designs and statistical tools in order to respond successfully to this challenge as up-to-date compliance monitoring provides information; this is simply too good an opportunity to ignore[1].

REFERENCES

1. Efron B. Foreword Limburg Compliance Symposium. *Stat Med* 1998;**17**:249–250.
2. Haynes RB. Introduction. In: Haynes RB, Taylor DW, Sackett DL eds. *Compliance in Health Care*. Baltimore: The Johns Hopkins University Press; 1979:1–7.
3. Dixon WM, Stradling P, Wootton IDP. Outpatient P.A.S. Therapy. *Lancet* 1957;**ii**:871–872.

4. Hasford J. Biometric Issues in Measuring and Analysing Partial Compliance in Clinical Trials. In: Cramer JA, Spilker B eds. *Patient Compliance in Medical Practice and Clinical Trials.* New York: Raven Press; 1991:265–281.

5. Psaty BM, Koepsell TD, Wagner EH, LoGerfo JP, Inui TS. The Relative Risk of Incident Coronary Heart Disease Associated With Recently Stopping the Use of b-Blockers. *JAMA* 1990;**263**:1653–1657.

6. Hasford J. Compliance and the Benefit/Risk Relationship of Antihypertensive Treatment. *J Cardiovasc Pharmacol* 1992;**20**(Suppl.6):S30–S34.

7. Cramer JA, Mattson RH. Monitoring Compliance with Antiepileptic Drug Therapy. In: Cramer JA, Spilker B eds. *Patient Compliance in Medical Practice and Clinical Trials.* New York: Raven Press; 1991:123–137.

8. Weis SE, Slocum PC, Blais FX, King B, Nunn M, Matney GB, Gomez E, Foresman BH. The Effect of Directly Observed Therapy on the Rates of Drug Resistance and Relapse in Tuberculosis. *N Engl J Med* 1994;**330**:1179–1184.

9. The Coronary Drug Project Group. Influence of Adherence to Treatment and Response of Cholesterol on Mortality in the Coronary Drug Project. *N Engl J Med* 1980;**303**:1038–1041.

10. Urquhart J, De Klerk E. Contending Paradigms For the Interpretation of Data on Patient Compliance with Therapeutic Drug Regimens. *Stat Med* 1998;**17**:251–267.

11. Cox D. Discussion. *Stat Med* 1998;**17**:387–389.

12. Gordis L, Markowitz M, Lilienfeld AM. Studies in the Epidemiology and Preventability of Rheumatic Fever. IV. A Quantitative Determination of Compliance in Children on Oral Penicillin Prophylaxis. *Pediatrics* 1969;**43**:173–182.

13. Haynes RB, McKibbon KA, Kanani R. Systematic Review of Randomised Trials of Interventions to Assist Patients to Follow Prescriptions for Medications. *Lancet* 1996;**348**:383–386.

14. Edmonds E, Förster E, Greminger P, Groth H, Siegenthaler W, Vetter W. Der Effekt der Blutdruckselbstmessung auf die Compliance des Hypertonikers. *Schweiz Rundsch Med Prax* 1985;**8**:173–176.

15. Probstfield JI. Clinical Trial Prerandomization Compliance (Adherence) Screen. In: Cramer JA, Spilker B eds. *Patient Compliance in Medical Practice and Clinical Trials.* New York: Raven Press;1991:323–333.

16. Schechtman KB, Gordon MO. The Effect of Poor Compliance and Treatment Side Effects on Sample Size Requirements in Randomized Clinical Trials. *J Biopharmaceut Stat* 1994;**4**:223–232.

17. Nived O, Sturfelt G, Eckernäs S, Singer P. A Comparison of 6 Months' Compliance of Patients with Rheumatoid Arthritis Treated with Tenoxicam and Naproxen. Use of Patient Computer Data to Assess Response to Treatment. *J Rheumatol* 1994;**21**:1537–1541.

18. Vrijens B, Goetghebeur EJT. Comparing Compliance Patterns Between Randomized Treatments. *Contr Clin Trials* 1997;**18**:187–203.

19. Sheiner LB, Rubin DB. Intention-to-treat analysis and the goals of clinical trials. *Clin Pharmacol Ther* 1994;**57**:6–15.

20. Efron B, Feldman D. Compliance as an Explanatory Variable in Clinical Trials. *J Am Stat Assoc* 1991;**86**:7–17.

21. Rubin DB. More Powerful Randomization-Based P-Values in Double-Blind Trials with Non-compliance. *Stat Med* 1998;**17**:371–385.

22. Goetghebeur EJT, Molenberghs G, Katz J. Estimating the Causal Effect of Compliance on Binary Outcome in Randomized Controlled Trials. *Stat Med* 1998;**17**:341–355.

23. White IR, Goetghebeur EJT. Clinical Trials Comparing Two Treatment Policies: Which Aspects of the Treatment Policies Make a Difference? *Stat Med* 1998;**17**:319–339.
24. Goetghebeur EJT, Pocock SJ. Statistical Issues In Allowing For Noncompliance And Withdrawal. *Drug Inform J* 1993;**27**:837–845.
25. Robins JM. Correction for Non-Compliance in Equivalence Trials. *Stat Med* 1998;**17**:269–302.
26. Lipid Research Clinic Program. The Lipid Research Clinics Coronary Primary Prevention Trial Results, Parts I and II. *JAMA* 1984;**251**:351–374.

3

Achieving and Assessing Therapeutic Coverage

Peter A. Meredith

Gardiner Institute, Western Infirmary, Glasgow, UK

INTRODUCTION

The potential problem of poor compliance with prescribed therapy has long been recognized. However, although prescribing physicians are prepared to concede that inadequate compliance with treatment regimens is widespread, it is not uncommon to encounter an attitude which suggests firstly that this pattern of behaviour does exist but not in their patients and secondly that, where it does exist, it is a reflection of aberrant behaviour. Clearly, both of these statements are incorrect. Indeed, the evidence suggests that the prevalence of inadequate compliance is in many instances so high as to suggest that it might be considered as a reflection of normal rather than aberrant behaviour. The somewhat naive attitudes to compliance that have been adopted in the past are, at least in part, due to findings in clinical trials where patients are studied and monitored in a relatively intense fashion which tends to sustain compliance at a high rate and where estimates of compliance in clinical trials are determined by returned tablet counts. The validity of the latter technique can now be seriously called into question and it is clear from studies reported elsewhere in this book that electronic monitoring provides a much more realistic insight into patterns of compliance in long-term, routine clinical practice.

The summarising data from these studies suggest that, whilst approximately one-third of patients are achieving a reasonable level of compliance (in excess of 80%), a substantial proportion of the population are suboptimal compliers and, indeed, a small number of patients are taking very little drug at all. Thus, it is now clear that the most common pattern of poor patient compliance is characterised by delayed dosing (by hours, sometimes by days and occasionally by weeks) and, in general, that this is followed by a resumption of full-strength dosing. This chapter will, therefore, focus upon the potential

Drug Regimen Compliance: Issues in Clinical Trials and Patient Management.
Edited by J.-M. Métry and U.A. Meyer. © 1999 John Wiley & Sons Ltd.

consequences of such patterns of suboptimal compliance and, in particular, to consider the characteristics of alternative therapies and their ability to compensate or 'forgive' these inadequacies in compliance.

HOW MUCH COMPLIANCE IS SUFFICIENT TO IMPROVE OUTCOME?

In many respects this is a question which has rarely been posed in therapeutics. Many physicians have simply assumed that there can be no compromise with a scientifically defined drug dosing regimen. However, it is important to appreciate that compliance, when appropriately defined, refers to the extent to which the time history of the patient's dosing corresponds to the prescribed regimen. Since the treatment regimen specifies both quantity and timing of doses, focusing only on the percentage of prescribed doses taken can lead to false conclusions about the therapeutic superiority of one drug treatment regimen over another. In this instance, the crucial matter is not the number or percentage of prescribed doses taken, but the continuity of therapeutic action. Different drugs differ in their abilities to 'forgive' errors in compliance by maintaining therapeutic action in the face of certain well established lapses in dosing. Thus, some therapeutic agents may demand punctual dosing in order to maintain action whereas others can maintain action when a dose is occasionally omitted or taken belatedly. Recognition of this fact has resulted in the development of the concept of therapeutic coverage.

THERAPEUTIC COVERAGE

Therapeutic coverage is the parameter that utilises information on a drug's pharmacodynamic duration of action, together with a profile of dosing history, and it reflects the percentage of time that the drug's action is sustained within an established therapeutic range[1]. The principles underlying this concept are illustrated in Figure 3.1, and it is apparent that by identifying the therapeutic coverage for a specific drug, it may be possible to design a drug regimen that can 'forgive' the most commonly occurring compliance error— namely, dosage omissions. Continuity of action and maintenance of therapeutic coverage is best ensured when the prescribed dosing interval between doses is substantially shorter than (preferably half or less) the duration of drug action. This principle applies irrespective of the frequency of dosing and can be exemplified by comparing the effects of taking a product at half the strength, twice daily, with taking the same produce once daily at full strength. With the twice-daily dosing regimen the formulation and pharmacodynamic characteristics of the drug will give each dose a duration of action of about

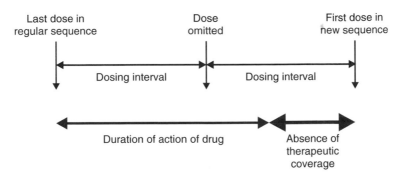

FIGURE 3.1 Principles underlying the concept of therapeutic coverage

24 hours, and it will not need to be taken on a strict 12–hourly basis but more conveniently at bedtime and on awakening, even though the interdose intervals will be unequal. If the occasional dose is omitted, drug action is able to continue, with at least half strength, until the time of the next scheduled dose—which, if taken, serves to maintain drug action. In this manner, the twice-daily regimen can achieve better continuity of drug action than the once-daily regimen, even if a few more doses are omitted from the twice-daily dosing regimen. This theoretical consideration finds support in a study comparing the antihypertensive efficacy of equal doses of enalapril administered either once or twice daily[2]. The twice-daily regimen not only produced smoother and more consistent blood pressure control but also offered superior therapeutic coverage of antihypertensive effect following a missed dose[2].

How to Achieve and Define Good Therapeutic Coverage

The treatment of cardiovascular disease (and, in particular, the treatment of hypertension) represents a useful model when considering the potential benefits of good therapeutic coverage and how to achieve it. Hypertension, even at mild to moderate levels, is associated with significant cardiovascular morbidity and mortality. However, it is a relatively asymptomatic disease and many patients show suboptimal compliance with antihypertensive treatment regimens. The results of the major intervention studies in hypertension confirm that antihypertensive therapy can reduce the risk of both stroke and coronary heart disease (CHD)[3]. The benefits of antihypertensive therapy were clearly demonstrated with regard to the reduction in stroke; however, although the epidemiological studies predict a reduction of up to 25% in CHD for a modest 6 mmHg reduction in diastolic blood pressure, the randomised outcome trials elicited only a 16% reduction. One likely explanation for this shortfall can be attributed to a relative therapeutic failure. Support for this assertion can be found in the documented failure of between one-quarter and one-third of patients to achieve the blood pressure control targets at the outset of most trials of antihypertensive treatment[4]. The therapeutic shortcomings in antihypertensive therapy have been recognised for some time in clinical practice[5] when mortality in 'controlled' hypertensives exceeded that in normotensive controls with similar clinic blood pressure measurements. Furthermore, recent studies assessing blood pressure control based upon ambulatory blood pressure monitoring have clearly demonstrated the therapeutic shortcomings of existing antihypertensive treatment regimens[6]. This latter study may also be indicative of a failure to achieve ideal blood pressure control, which should, upon epidemiological evidence, be based upon strategies that lower blood pressure consistently and fully throughout 24 hours[7].

It is apparent, therefore, that there is considerable scope for improving therapeutic strategies in the treatment of hypertension. It is also clear that, when designing rational therapeutic regimens for the treatment of this condition, it is important to have some insight into the therapeutic coverage offered by any given agent. Insight into a drug's therapeutic coverage may be derived indirectly from observational studies. Figure 3.2 illustrates the correlation of blood pressure response to once-daily administration of nitrendipine, with the rates of compliance assessed by electronic monitoring[8]. The authors of this particular study noted a negative linear correlation between blood pressure response and rate of compliance. However, it is more important to note that, on a group basis, levels of compliance must be sustained above 90% in order to achieve a fall in blood pressure with a once-daily treatment regimen of nitrendipine. By inference, it can be concluded that this agent, when administered once daily, has a relatively modest duration of action and can achieve blood pressure control only when adherence to the treatment

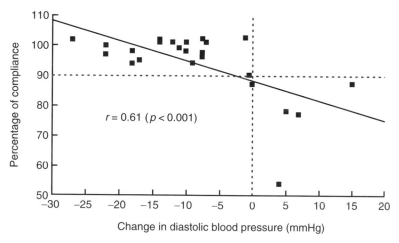

FIGURE 3.2 The correlation of blood pressure response to nitrendipine once daily and the rate of compliance assessed using electronic monitoring

regimen is relatively high. An alternative interpretation could be that the drug has a very limited ability to maintain antihypertensive efficacy in the setting of poor compliance, and thus can be regarded as having poor therapeutic coverage.

A second indirect method for assessing therapeutic coverage depends upon clinical observation in individual patients related to precise measures of compliance in that patient. This was exemplified by the study of Rudd[9] with respect to the apparent secondary resistance to antihypertensive treatment in a patient who, initially, responded favourably to treatment. Figure 3.3 shows the data for a patient who underwent a placebo washout for a month before starting antihypertensive therapy with twice-daily isradipine. The upper panel shows a good blood pressure response, beginning after 2 months' participation in the study, but disappears by the last visit. An indirect measure of compliance, based upon tablet counts, illustrates satisfactory adherence to the treatment regimen in the 91–108% range. Neither the prescribed daily dose nor the dose actually administered in the 24 hours before the scheduled visit correlated well with changes in systolic blood pressure. The lower panel highlights the critical parameter: the interval between the last administered dose and the clinical assessment of blood pressure. The best blood pressure response was apparent when the dosage interval was relatively short (0.8–3 hours on days 75 and 90), but antihypertensive control was lost on the final visit when the dosage interval rose above 10 hours. The authors concluded that the patient's apparent resistance to antihypertensive therapy was likely to be secondary to lapses in medication taking rather than to biological or pharmacological resistance[8].

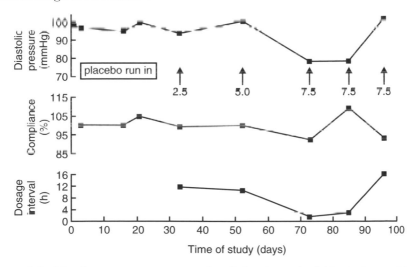

Figure 3.3 Blood pressure response to isradipine in an individual along with two measures of compliance. Arrows indicate dose of isradipine given per day. See text for further details

Direct Assessment of Therapeutic Coverage

The direct, and almost certainly most appropriate, method for assessing therapeutic coverage is to evaluate the duration of action of antihypertensive drugs from studies that deliberately mimic the most commonly observed pattern of poor treatment compliance (dosage omissions or belated dosing). Such studies have been performed in the past, though not necessarily with the aim of defining therapeutic coverage, rather the aim was to demonstrate that a particular therapeutic agent did not exhibit any 'rebound' effects following withdrawal of therapy. For example, a study performed with bopindolol[10] was designed to examine blood pressure responses following withdrawal of a beta-blocker to exclude the possibility of 'rebound' or 'overshoot' hypertension. The results of this study are summarised in Table 3.1 and the authors suggested that there was no evidence for safety concerns, with regard to the development of excessive rises in blood pressure, following withdrawal of treatment. However, it is apparent from Table 3.1 that, perhaps more importantly, there was little or no maintenance of any antihypertensive efficacy following withdrawal of treatment in that the systolic and diastolic blood pressures 1 day after stopping treatment were comparable to the blood pressures 1–2 weeks later. This suggests that bopindolol will not offer particularly effective therapeutic coverage in the face of even a single 'missed dose'.

More recently, 'missed dose' studies have been performed with the specific aim of characterising the therapeutic coverage of different agents. For example, a randomised controlled trial compared the antihypertensive efficacy and duration of response to once-daily beta-adrenoceptor antagonists (betaxolol and atenolol) by deliberately substituting a placebo for active drug on one of the steady-state treatment days[11]. The different agents were compared on the basis of ambulatory blood pressure responses, both with active steady-state treatment and following the insertion of the placebo dose. With active treatment, the antihypertensive effects and safety profiles of the two agents were comparable. However, following withdrawal of treatment the maintenance of antihypertensive effect was very different for the two drugs (Figure 3.4). The 24-hour blood pressure profiles for betaxolol were comparable on

TABLE 3.1 Blood pressure responses to bopindolol following withdrawal of steady-state therapy

	Active treatment	Days after withdrawal of steady-state therapy		
		1	3	14
Systolic pressure (mmHg)	128 ± 10	143 ± 12	142 ± 8	143 ± 6
Diastolic pressure (mmHg)	84 ± 4	93 ± 6	97 ± 4	95 ± 2
Heart rate (beats/min)	63 ± 4	66 ± 4	70 ± 3	70 ± 3

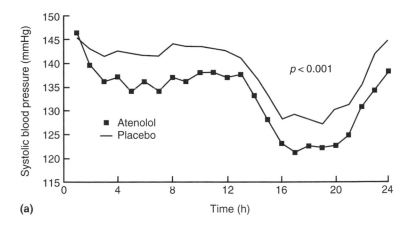

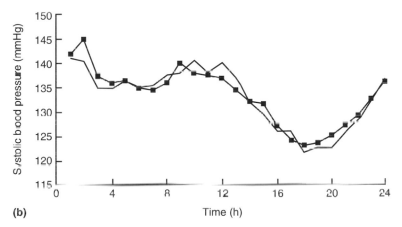

Figure 3.4 The ambulatory blood pressure responses to once-daily therapy with (a) atenolol and (b) betaxolol: the effect of a single 'missed dose' (placebo profile)

active treatment and placebo days; in contrast, the effect of atenolol rapidly diminished following withdrawal of treatment, such that the blood pressures were statistically significantly higher than those observed during active treatment, as assessed by analysis of variance ($p < 0.001$). Thus, it is clear that with precise dosing and good treatment adherence the antihypertensive efficacy of atenolol and betaxolol are comparable but that, in contrast, the drugs differ significantly with respect to their therapeutic coverage and that betaxolol is clearly superior in this instance. In pharmacological terms, both agents have similar properties, being cardioselective beta-blockers. However, significant differences in the disposition characteristics of these two agents are characterised by the longer elimination half-life of betaxolol, indicating that the differences in therapeutic coverage may be associated with their pharmacokinetic characteristics.

Therapeutic Coverage and Pharmacokinetic Characteristics

There is a widely held (and largely anecdotal) view that there is no relationship between the plasma concentration of an antihypertensive drug and its blood pressure lowering effect, but a volume of evidence suggests that this view is in fact largely incorrect. A substantial volume of data from a wide range of different antihypertensive agents indicates that, where a study has been appropriately conducted and analysed, it is possible to integrate pharmacokinetic and pharmacodynamic indices to characterise a mathematical description of blood pressure response in individual patients. Thus, relationships can be identified between drug concentrations and antihypertensive effect[12]. However, it is also clear that the correlations are not always direct and may be compromised by a temporal discrepancy between the concentration and effect profiles. Furthermore, the exact mathematical relationship between the circulating drug concentration and the elicited effect may determine the duration of action of the drug and thus its therapeutic coverage[13].

Pharmacokinetic/Pharmacodynamic Interrelationships

The importance of the pharmacokinetic characteristics and the exact nature of the concentration–effect relationship can be demonstrated by considering two alternative and theoretical antihypertensive agents (Figure 3.5). Although both drugs achieve the same maximum concentration (Figure 3.5(a)), the drug with the longer half-life (A) has higher concentrations at trough and smaller fluctuations in concentrations over the steady-state dosage interval. In contrast, the antihypertensive response profiles for these two agents are broadly comparable (Figure 3.5(b)); indeed, the blood pressure reductions at peak and trough can be superimposed. If these two agents were alternative candidates for development as antihypertensive agents it would not be possible, on the basis of the trough and peak blood pressure responses, to offer any opinion as to which would offer significant advantage with respect to therapeutic coverage. The trough to peak ratio of blood pressure response has been proposed by the licensing authorities as an index of the duration of action of an antihypertensive drug[14]. It would therefore not be unusual in characterising a new agent to determine not only the dose–response relationship but also the influence of dose upon the trough:peak ratio. From the data derived for drugs A and B (Table 3.2) it is clear that, despite the fact that these two agents have similar effect profiles when administered at a dose of 20 mg once daily, the dose–response relationships are disparate and the trough:peak ratio for drug B is much more dose dependent than it is for drug A. At a superficial level, it might be argued that it would be difficult to explain the apparent discrepancy between these agents on the basis of a pharmacokinetic/pharmacodynamic (PK/PD) relationship. In reality these results are entirely explicable on the basis of the pharmacokinetics of the two drugs and the concentration–effect relationship (Figure 3.6). The differences between the two drugs are related to their exact concentration–effect relationship, such that for drug A the concentrations achieved with the selected doses are all less than the CE_{50} value, and thus the concentration–effect relationship is relatively linear: in contrast, with drug B, in many instances the concentrations exceed the drug concentration producing 50% of the maximal response (CE_{50}) and thus the concentration–effect relationship conforms much more to the non-linear or F_{max}-type relationship (curvilinear relationship that defines the theoretical maximal response).

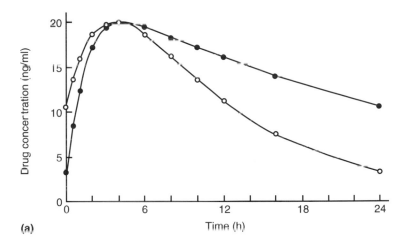

(a)

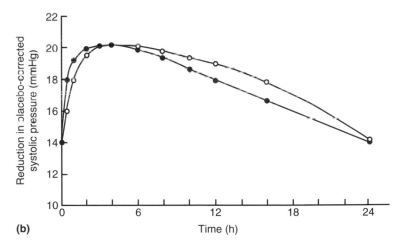

(b)

FIGURE 3.5   (a) The steady-state pharmacokinetic profile of two hypothetical drugs: A (●) and B (○). (b) The steady-state antihypertensive response to the two drugs

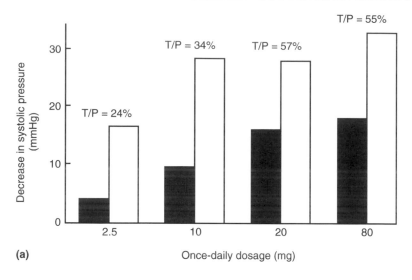

(a)

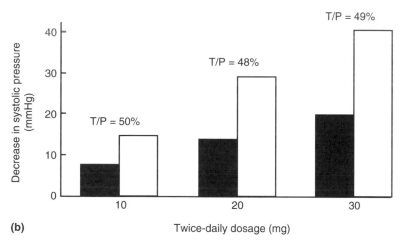

(b)

FIGURE 3.6 The dose–response relationship at peak (□) and trough (■) for lisinopril, administered once daily (a) and nifedipine retard, administered twice daily (b)

TABLE 3.2 Trough:peak response to different doses of two hypothetical antihypertensive drugs

	Dose (mg)			
	2.5	5	10	20
Drug A	45%	48%	52%	59%
Drug B	30%	37%	46%	59%

These hypothetical considerations have been demonstrated in clinical studies. For example, the dose–response relationship and the effect of dose on trough:peak ratio with lisinopril are quite different from those seen with nifedipine[15] (Figure 3.6). Formal concentration–effect analysis indicates that for angiotensin-converting enzyme (ACE) inhibitors such as lisinopril the concentration–effect relationship is indeed of the E_{max} type whilst for nifedipine and other dihydropyridine calcium antagonists, the relationship is essentially linear[12]. It may thus be reasonably concluded that the pharmacokinetic characteristics and the exact concentration–effect relationship will determine the profile of action of an antihypertensive drug. Furthermore, it may again be reasonably concluded that these relationships will also determine the therapeutic coverage of a pharmacological agent and its therapeutic regimen.

The Importance of Concentration–Effect Relationships in Determining Therapeutic Coverage

If consideration is given once again to the theoretical agents A and B, it would be anticipated that the differences would become even more apparent when the concentration and effect profiles are studied beyond the end of the dosage interval. Figure 3.7 shows the concentration profile for both drugs over a 48-hour period at steady state, assuming a 'missed dose' at 24 hours and the corresponding blood pressure profile. These figures highlight the fact that the difference between the two agents increases in the face of a 'missed dose', where drug A sustains its effect much less efficiently than drug B. These theoretical considerations are supported by data derived from clinical studies.

This study directly compared the ACE inhibitor enalapril and the hydropyridine calcium antagonist amlodipine. Both are deemed to be suitable for once-daily administration and both achieve trough:peak ratios for blood pressure response in excess of 50%. However, the drugs differ in pharmacokinetics and PK/PD relationships. The half-life of amlodipine is approximately 48 hours and the PK/PD is essentially linear. In contrast, the accumulation half-life for enalapril is approximately 12 hours and the PK/PD is of the E_{max} type. The 'missed dose' study[16] was carried out in 30 hypertensive patients, divided into two groups who, after an initial 4-week placebo run-in period, were treated with either amlodipine (5 mg once daily) or enalapril (20 mg once daily) for 12 weeks. Ambulatory blood pressure monitoring was undertaken at the end of the placebo run-in phase, during the active steady-state treatment regiment, and after missing one daily dose. The results are summarised in Figure 3.8. It is immediately apparent that, whilst following a 'missed dose', amlodipine in the main sustains its antihypertensive effect relative to active treatment, with enalapril there was a gradual diminution of effect such that in the period 16–24 hours after a 'missed dose' its

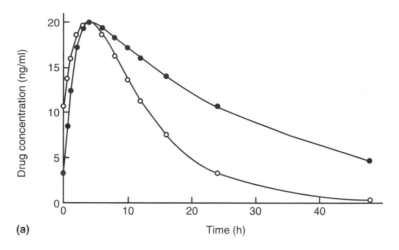

(a)

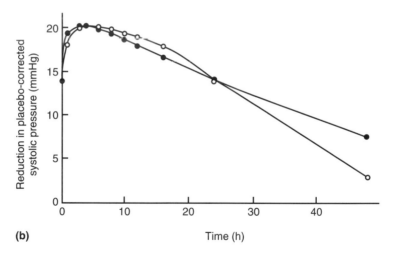

(b)

FIGURE 3.7 The pharmacokinetic profile of (a) two hypothetical antihypertensive agents A (●) and B (○) at steady state over a 48-hour period, and (b) the equivalent placebo-corrected blood pressure profile, following a 'missed dose'

antihypertensive effect is virtually lost. Thus, whilst both drugs reduced systolic and diastolic blood pressure during steady-state treatment, when patients missed a dose of enalapril control of blood pressure was progressively lost. In contrast, blood pressure of patients taking amlodipine was controlled over the full 24 hours of a 'missed dosage' interval.

Although the pharmacokinetic characteristics of a drug and the concentration–effect relationship are important determinants of therapeutic coverage, it should also be appreciated that the pharmacological potency of

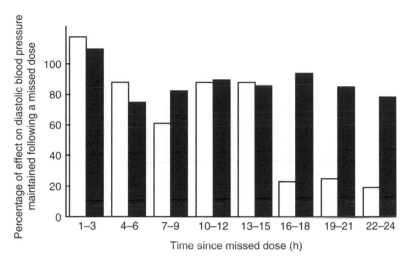

FIGURE 3.8 Maintenance of the antihypertensive response to amlodipine (■) and enalapril (□) following the insertion of a 'missed dose' into a steady-state treatment regimen

different agents will also play an important role. This can be highlighted by consideration of a study which directly compared the two ACE inhibitors trandolapril and enalapril in a 'missed dose' study. These agents have similar pharmacokinetic properties, their concentration–effect relationships are of the E_{max} type and the clinical blood pressure responses were broadly comparable for the doses selected in this study. However, the haemodynamic profiles of these two agents, as assessed by ambulatory blood pressure monitoring, are distinctly different (Figure 3.9). Trandolapril achieves a much higher trough:peak ratio for blood pressure response than enalapril and sustains this effect despite a 'missed dose'[17].

Assessing Extended Therapeutic Coverage

The implications of the theoretical considerations detailed earlier in this chapter, and supported by practical clinical studies, are that for an antihypertensive drug the blood pressure response is most likely to be sustained where circulating drug concentrations are maintained at a relatively consistent level over a steady-state dosage interval, and where the relationship between concentration in effect is relatively linear. One might, therefore, anticipate that a drug with an intrinsically long half-life should not only achieve optimal blood pressure control in terms of a smooth and consistent blood pressure lowering effect but also offer good therapeutic coverage, with an effect sustained well beyond the end of the dosage interval. In pharmacokinetic terms amlodipine appears to approach this 'ideal' characteristic. In a study that was specifically

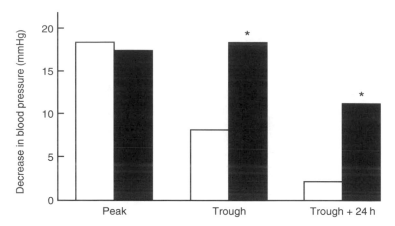

FIGURE 3.9 The peak and trough blood pressure responses to trandolapril (2 mg twice daily; ■) and enalapril (20 mg once daily; □) and the response 24 hours after a 'missed dose'. $*p<0.01$ compared with enalapril

designed to establish whether there was a close relationship between the pharmacokinetics of amlodipine and its antihypertensive effect[18], a close correlation was observed between plasma drug concentration and blood pressure lowering effect (Figure 3.10). Not only is it apparent that the antihypertensive effect at steady-state is superimposed relatively consistently upon the blood pressure response, measured under placebo conditions, but it is also apparent that there is little diminution in the antihypertensive response to amlodipine even 48 hours after the dose.

This, and the earlier study described[16], implies that amlodipine has sufficient therapeutic coverage to compensate for a single dosage omission.

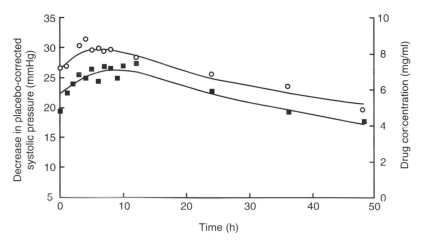

FIGURE 3.10 Concentration (○) and placebo-corrected systolic blood pressure response (■) to amlodipine in a representative hypertensive patient

However, based upon its pharmacokinetic characteristics and its established concentration–effect relationship, it would be anticipated that amlodipine would have a therapeutic coverage in excess of 48 hours, and might be capable of maintaining a useful blood pressure lowering effect when more than one dose is omitted. This possibility has been examined by comparison of amlodipine, which is a calcium antagonist with a long elimination half-life, and diltiazem, a calcium antagonist with a short elimination half-life[19]. In this study, the blood pressure lowering effect of both drugs was assessed by 24-hour ambulatory blood pressure monitoring, both on active maintenance treatment and after treatment was interrupted for 2 days by placebo (using a double-blind, randomised design). After a single-blind placebo run-in period, hypertensive patients were randomised to amlodipine (5 mg once daily) or diltiazem (90 mg twice daily). After 4–6 weeks of therapy, the doses were increased to 10 mg once daily or 180 mg twice daily, if necessary, for control of diastolic blood pressure. During maintenance therapy the blood pressure responses to amlodipine and diltiazem were comparable (Figure 3.11(a)). In contrast, the persistence of the antihypertensive response after insertion of 2 days of placebo treatment differed for the two different agents (Figure 3.11(b)). It is clear that the antihypertensive effect of amlodipine clearly persisted (none of the differences between the active and interrupted treatment was statistically significant). In contrast, only a small antihypertensive effect was observed with diltiazem during the day compared with the blood pressure at the end of the placebo run-in period; by night, the effect had been almost totally abolished (Figure 3.11). Based upon the ambulatory blood pressure monitoring approach adopted in this study it would appear that, whilst amlodipine and diltiazem produce similar antihypertensive effects during fully compliant maintenance treatment, during a short period of non-compliance the blood pressure control was better with the agent with the long elimination half-life (amlodipine) than with the agent with short elimination half-life (diltiazem). Analysis of data from this study[20] provided an additional insight into the therapeutic coverage provided by the different agents. Patients were arbitrarily divided on the basis of whether their compliance exceeded or was less than 80%, using the percentage of prescribed doses actually taken measured by electronic monitoring. The results are summarised in Figure 3.12. In patients treated with amlodipine compliance was not a determinant of blood pressure control but for patients treated with diltiazem, when compliance was less than 80% the blood pressure reduction was approximately half that achieved by patients with a compliance rate in excess of 80%.

INTRINSIC LONG DURATION OF ACTION VERSUS FORMULATION

As discussed earlier, our current understanding of the pathogenesis of hypertension-related disease appears to favour the use of long-acting

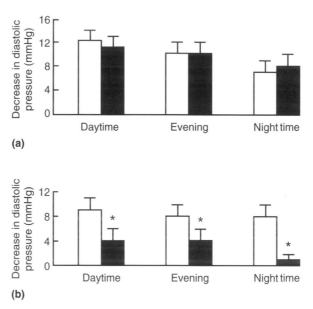

(a)

(b)

Figure 3.11 The diastolic blood pressure responses to amlodipine (■) and diltiazem (□) assessed by ambulatory monitoring during maintenance therapy (a) and following two days of placebo ('non-compliant' patient) (b). Bars represent standard deviation; *$p<0.05$

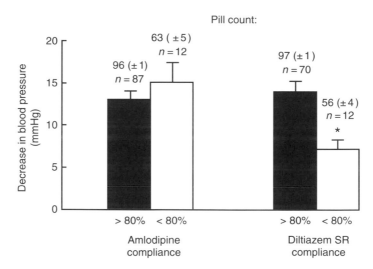

Figure 3.12 The clinical blood pressure responses to amlodipine and diltiazem during maintenance therapy with an arbitrary subdivision of patients, based upon whether their compliance was greater or less than 80%. Bars represent standard deviation; *$p<0.05$

antihypertensive agents that provide smooth and consistent antihypertensive effect over a steady-state dosing interval. This can be achieved either by using agents that have intrinsic long duration of action or by the use of drugs which have been subject to pharmaceutical manipulation and reformulated using sophisticated formulation approaches. The benefits of reformulating a drug can clearly be demonstrated with nifedipine[21]. Table 3.3 summarises the results of a randomised parallel group comparison of the long-acting formulation of nifedipine (nifedipine GITS) administered once daily with nifedipine SR, which is administered twice daily. The sophisticated reformulated once-per-day formulation offers significant benefit, not only with respect to three different measures of compliance with the treatment regimen but also in terms of improved blood pressure control.

Although long-acting formulations may, over a steady-state dosage interval, mimic the plasma concentration profile of an intrinsically long-acting agent, caution must be exercised in considering that the formulation-dependent drug will offer the same therapeutic coverage as an alternative agent with a long elimination half-life. From first principles it would be anticipated that following one or more missed doses a discrimination would be possible between the intrinsically long-acting agent, where the drug's effect would be sustained, and the formulation-dependent drug, where the effect will diminish rapidly once the formulation has been exhausted. This is apparent in a direct comparison of the antihypertensive effects of amlodipine and nifedipine GITS[22], where the achieved blood pressure control, as assessed by ambulatory daytime diastolic blood pressures, is essentially comparable (Figure 3.13). Following a single missed dose the blood pressure response to amlodipine is sustained but missing a dose of nifedipine GITS causes the blood pressure to rise slightly and statistically significant differences become apparent between the two different agents (as assessed by analysis of variance). The substantial difference in the antihypertensive efficacy of these agents becomes apparent following two missed doses: once again, the blood

TABLE 3.3 Blood pressure responses and compliance rates with once-daily nifedipine GITS and twice-daily nifedipine SR

	Nifedipine GITS	Nifedipine SR
Pill count	104 ± 4	93 ± 2
MEMS compliance:		
Prescribed doses taken (%)	93*	84
Days with correct number of doses (%)	87*	72
Doses taken on time (%)	70*	50
Blood pressure response (%)	82*	59

*$p<0.01$. Responders defined as patients with >80% compliance and who achieve blood pressure control by virtue of diastolic pressure >90 mmHg or with a fall in diastolic pressure of more than 10 mmHg

pressure with amlodipine is similar to that seen with full compliance, whereas with nifedipine GITS there is a statistically significant ($p<0.01$) and clinically relevant loss of antihypertensive effect (Figure 3.13).

CONCLUSION

It is now clear that poor compliance in a wide range of therapeutic areas is more prevalent than previously recognised. In particular, poor compliance is often characterised by serial dosage omissions or 'drug holidays'. The implications of 'drug holidays' are particularly apparent in the treatment of hypertension and other cardiovascular diseases. Whilst the emphasis in improving compliance by patient education must remain, it is more realistic, and ultimately of greater clinical relevance, to select drugs and dosage regimens which can provide good therapeutic coverage despite dosage omissions. The different agents licensed for once-daily administration clearly differ in their therapeutic coverage, and this has been highlighted by studies that have deliberately sought to mimic patterns of poor compliance by inserting placebo doses into active steady-state treatment regimens. It is clear from these studies that (as would be anticipated from first principles) agents with prolonged elimination half-lives and a relatively linear correlation between drug concentration and effect are most likely to offer better therapeutic coverage.

Thus, the challenge in therapeutics is to define sufficiency. In this regard, therapeutic sufficiency with any given drug and treatment regimen will be defined by determining the level of medication taking that is sufficient to

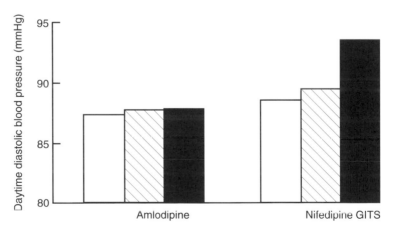

Figure 3.13 The blood pressure responses to amlodipine (5 mg once daily) and nifedipine GITS (30 mg once daily) during maintenance therapy (□) and following the insertion of one (▨) or two (■) days of placebo into the steady-state treatment regimen

produce the desired clinical effect as opposed to seeking to achieve perfect concordance with the prescribed dosage regimen.

REFERENCES

1. Urquhart J: Partial compliance in cardiovascular disease: risk implications. *Br J Clin Pract* 1994; **73:** 2–12.
2. Meredith PA, Donnelly R, Elliott HL, Howie CA and Reid JL: Prediction of the antihypertensive response to enalapril. *J Hypertens* 1990; **8:** 1085–1090.
3. Collins R and Peto R: Antihypertensive drug therapy: effects on stroke and coronary heart disease. In: *Textbook of Hypertension.* pp. 1156–1164. Swales JD (ed.). Blackwell Scientific Publications, Oxford, 1994.
4. Menard J: Improving hypertension treatment: where should we put our efforts—new drugs, new concepts or new management? *Am J Hypertens* 1992; **5:** 252S–258S.
5. Isles CG, Walker LM, Beevers GD, Brown I, Cameron HL, Clarke J, Hawthorne V, *et al*: Mortality of patients of the Glasgow Blood Pressure Clinic. *J Hypertens* 1986; **4:** 141–156.
6. Mancia G, Sega R, Milesi C, Cesana G and Zanchetti A: Blood pressure control in the hypertensive population. *Lancet* 1997; **349:** 454–457.
7. Meredith PA, Perloff D, Mancia G and Pickering T: Blood pressure variability and its implications for antihypertensive therapy. *Blood Pressure* 1995; **4:** 5–11.
8. Mallion JM, Meilhac B, Tremel F, Calvez R and Bertholom N: Use of a microprocessor-equipped tablet box in monitoring compliance with antihypertensive treatment. *J Cardiovasc Pharmacol* 1992; **19:** (Suppl 2): S41–S48.
9. Rudd P: Partial compliance: implications for clinical practice. *J Cardiovasc Pharmacol* 1993; **22:** S1–S5.
10. Bolli P, Amann FW, Muller FB, Meyer B, Burckhardt D and Buhler FR: Withdrawal of the long-acting beta-blocker, bopindolol, is not associated with beta-adrenoceptor super-sensitivity. *J Cardiovasc Pharmacol* 1986; **8:** (Suppl 6): S64–S69.
11. Johnson BF and Whelton A: A study design for comparing the effects of missing daily doses of antihypertensive drugs. *Am J Ther* 1994; **1:** 260–267.
12. Reid JL and Meredith PA: The use of pharmacodynamic and pharmacokinetic profiles in drug development for planning individual therapy. In: *Hypertension: Pathophysiology, Diagnosis and Management.* 2nd ed. pp. 2771–2783. Laragh JH, Brenner BM (eds). Raven Press, New York, 1995.
13. Levy G: A pharmacokinetic perspective on medicament non-compliance. *Clin Pharmacol Ther* 1993; **54:** 242–244.
14. Meredith PA and Elliott HL: FDA guidelines on trough:peak ratios in the evaluation of antihypertensive agents. *J Cardiovasc Pharmacol* 1994; **23:** S26–S30.
15. Meredith PA and Elliott HL: Concentration–effect relationships and implications for trough:peak ratio. *Am J Hypertens* 1996; **9:** 87S–90S.
16. Hernandez-Hernandez R, de Hernandez MJ, Armas-Padilla MC, Carvajal AR and Guerrero-Pajuelo J: The effects of missing a dose of enalapril versus amlodipine on ambulatory blood pressure. *Blood Pressure Monitoring* 1996; **1:** 121–126.
17. Vaur L, Dutrey-Dupagne C, Boussac J, Genes N, Bouvier d'Yvoire M, Elkik F and Meredith PA: Differential effects of a 'missed dose' of trandolapril and enalapril on blood pressure control in hypertensive patients. *J Cardiovasc Pharmacol* 1995; **26:** (1): 127–131.

18. Donnelly R, Meredith PA, Miller SHK, Howie CA and Elliott HL: Pharmacodynamic modelling of the antihypertensive response to amlodipine. *Clin Pharmacol Ther* 1993; **54:** (3): 303–310.
19. Leenen FHH, Fourney A, Notman G and Tanner J: Persistence of antihypertensive effect after 'missed doses' of calcium antagonist with long (amlodipine) versus short (diltiazem) elimination half-life. *Br J Clin Pharmacol* 1996; **41:** 83–88.
20. Leenen FHH, Wilson TW, Bolli P, Larochelle P, Myers M, Handa SP, Boileau G and Tanner J: (in collaboration with 20 family physicians): Patterns of compliance with once versus twice daily antihypertensive drug therapy in primary care: a randomised clinical trial, using electronic monitoring. *Can J Cardiol* 1997; **13:** 1–7.
21. Toal CB and Laplante L: Is there a difference in hypertensive patient compliance between a once a day or twice a day nifedipine? *Am J Hypertens* 1995; **8:** (4): (Part 2): D17.
22. Elliott HL and Meredith PA: The effect of missed doses on the antihypertensive responses to amlodipine and nifedipine GITS. *Clin Pharmacol Ther* 1998 (in press).

4

Modeling and Simulation of Variable Drug Exposure

Erik de Klerk

Department of Rheumatology, University Hospital Maastricht, The Netherlands

INTRODUCTION

Electronic monitoring (EM) of variable patient compliance consists of a system where, with the aid of microprocessor technology, time and date of opening of drug package are recorded and stored. The assumption that these time series of openings reflect actual drug intake is widely accepted[1-5]. This system has several advantages over 'traditional' measures of compliance such as pill counts, interview techniques, diaries or physician estimates[6].

- First, the measurement is much more precise and comprehensive: the data consist of time histories of dosing, which do not limit the information to a summary over the whole study period. Selected information can be summarized and compared, for example the week before the clinical visit of interest or weekdays compared with weekends.
- Second, it is much more difficult for a patient to censor or otherwise manipulate EM data; they must do so every day of the monitored period, while censoring of pill counts or diaries is very easy since the evidence of omitted doses can be hidden in one simple act (by emptying the medicine bottle). Pullar[7] gave a striking example of patients censoring their compliance data. He compared pill counts with chemical marker data, and concluded that pill counts 'grossly overestimates patient compliance'
- Finally, EM has the unique advantage of providing real-time compliance monitoring, for it gives the day-by-day compliance accurately, showing the full range of drug exposure as it integrates into the patterns of the patient's daily life. None of the traditional techniques can do this.

A full description of the method and its advantages and disadvantages can be found elsewhere[8].

Drug Regimen Compliance: Issues in Clinical Trials and Patient Management.
Edited by J.-M. Métry and U.A. Meyer. © 1999 John Wiley & Sons Ltd.

EM produces a large amount of data, necessitating the use of summary variables. Several variables have been used for this purpose[5,9,10,11], each with its own specific advantages and disadvantages. It is therefore necessary that an appropriate method of data summarization is chosen, depending largely on the goal and the setting of the analyses (which should be considered and specified beforehand). Summarization variables that take specific advantage of EM data include the percentage of days on which dosing occurred as prescribed and the percentage of days on which dosing deviated from that prescribed (under- or overdosing), which are particularly useful to describe the adequacy of drug intake and spacing between doses in trials[11]. Another example is time variability in drug intake[9], which is special because it accounts for timing of drug intake and does not mask 'no-dose' days by 'catch-up' double dosing. A third example is the frequency histogram of interdose intervals[12], which shows the (often markedly skewed) deviation from the optimal interdose interval.

Drug holidays, arbitrarily defined as periods of three or more consecutive days without dosing[13], deserve special interest in many compliance-related analyses. Depending on the drug and the disease, drug holidays can lead to problems such as loss of efficacy[14,15], safety problems[16] (rebound effects and first-dose effect or emergence of resistant organisms in antimicrobial treatment[17]), or misattribution of side-effects[18].

One of the lessons of a decade of studies with electronic monitoring[8] is the remarkable similarity in variable compliance between different diseases, drugs and settings[3,5,9,19–21]. If this general distribution holds true for most trials, which seems to be approximately true although exceptions will doubtless emerge, this 'non-compliance likeliness' seems to be at least as important in determining the observed compliance as the occurrence of side-effects, feedback mechanisms on the drugs' effectiveness, and the amount of knowledge the patient has on his or her disease, drug, and prognosis.

Looking at a distribution of drug holidays[22], a question that easily arises is: is it possible to identify patients, from a limited period of measurement, who are likely to be frequent drug holiday takers? Such identification could then be used, for example, as a prerandomization variable, as a basis for stratified randomization in smaller trials, or as a basis for selective study of the effects of particular patterns of recurring non-compliance to enhance the comparability between study groups.

The often-used variable 'percentage of prescribed doses taken' is not accurate enough as a summary measure to be used as a stratification variable. If, for example, a patient has taken 85% of all doses during a 3-month measurement period, he or she could still have taken one 14-day drug holiday, two 7-day drug holidays, or 14 1-day omissions. The impact of the pattern of variable dosing will vary with the drug (contemplate, as an example, the impact of the variable patterns between oral contraceptives, non-ISA beta-blockers, digoxin, tamoxifen, antibiotics or analgesic NSAIDs). To further demonstrate the inaccuracy of 'percentage of prescribed doses taken' as a summary measure we took the average compliance, defined as the percentage of prescribed doses taken, as the probability of taking the next dose and compared the expected frequency of drug holidays with the observed number of drug holidays in a trial comparing two NSAIDs for ankylosing spondylitis (Figure 4.1) (trial methodology and results have been described in detail elsewhere[11,22]).

Figure 4.1 clearly depicts the large difference between the number of short drug holidays expected when we take the 'pill count' as predicting the variable, versus the observed, frequency of drug holidays. With drug holidays of longer duration, which are usually clinically most relevant, the variable does not appear to have any useful predictive potential. Yet this 'number of doses taken' is the most widely reported variable in the literature on patient compliance, even in papers using FM. We believe better variables must be defined. There are hundreds of possibilities. To examine the potential of each individual variable, and combinations of variables we propose the use of computer simulation.

SIMULATION

Simulation may be described as a means of organizing knowledge in a dynamic form that allows projections of this knowledge, sometimes revealing contradictions between the projections and reality. A logical next step is to

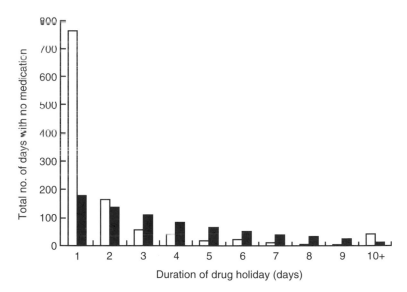

FIGURE 4.1 Difference between observed (☐) and expected (■) frequency of drug holidays when using percentage of prescribed doses taken as probability to take the next dose

identify the sources of any contradictions and devise a way to resolve them. In this sense simulation is conceptually no different than the scientific method, which searches for contradictions or inconsistencies between what is believed and what is observed.

Simulation has proven to be a powerful tool in many situations, a recent and stunning example of which was the development of the Boeing 777. The development of the plane was staged: first computer models were used to design individual parts, then the different parts were integrated into a larger model to simulate their behavior under diverse operating conditions in order to identify, anticipate and resolve potential problems before developing the first flying test model. The technique ensured rapid, efficient development and saved millions of dollars. The subsequent performance of the plane in daily operation has borne out the expectation that design by simulation would minimize risk and optimize the plane's performance characteristics.

Developing a Model

In order to estimate the effect of variable compliance upon efficacy of a drug one must start by considering the patterns in which compliance may vary, and estimate the patterns of variable compliance that may 'hurt' the drug. For example, the approach to an antibiotic which has to be taken for 7 days but which is usually effective when used correctly for 4 days will be different from that to a drug like a non-ISA beta-blocker that is harmful when intake is interrupted for more than 3 but less than 7 days. Rank ordering patients by percentage of doses taken, and describing various aspects of drug holidays in a spreadsheet format[22] can be used as a starting point, incorporating both frequency and duration of drug holidays as variables in the model.

If real compliance data are available, for example from a pilot study or a run-in period, they can serve as a starting point. Otherwise it is useful to start with a hypothetical distribution of usual compliance following the rule of sixes, or a hypothetical distribution of all possible patterns of interdose intervals, for example described in a rank-ordered spreadsheet format[22].

Considerations that must be taken into account will usually be drug specific, depending on pharmacokinetic and pharmacodynamic properties, and disease specific, depending on disease mechanism, the site of interaction of the drug with the disease and whether the disease is acute or chronic. Although the principles are the same, the specifics will differ with each situation. The potential hazards of variable compliance include loss of efficacy (e.g. by skipping doses of oral contraceptives), increase of hazards (e.g. loss of antiepileptic action), hazardous rebound effects (e.g. unblocked upregulated beta receptors upon cessation of non-ISA beta-blockers), and first-dose effects after dose restarts (e.g. following a drug holiday from nifedipine).

It is then possible to create a mathematical model that accepts optimal and various suboptimal patterns of drug intake as input, perhaps incorporate the pharmacokinetic and pharmacodynamic properties of the drug, and/or estimate the efficacy of the drug and the prevalence of the unwanted effects of variable compliance. The individual variables and parameters of the model, and the defined relationships between the variables, will differ from drug to drug.

The first example of a model that used electronic monitoring compliance data to make pharmacometric predictions was provided by Rubio et al[23]. These investigators used a model of diltiazem pharmacokinetics to project plasma levels of the drug under the assumption that intake was optimal (i.e. as prescribed). They then used the EM data, incorporating actual time histories of dosing of diltiazem as input, and projected the actual plasma concentrations. They reported data for four selected patients, showing that different patterns of variable compliance had a very different impact on the plasma levels reached. This information raised the question of how the different patterns of dosing have different impacts on plasma levels (and presumably also on clinical correlates).

Girard et al. defined a Markov model[10], which estimates compliance based on the assumption that the probability of taking a dose depends only on the number of doses associated with the previous nominal dosing interval. Analyses of simulations indicated that traditional population pharmacokinetic analysis methods that ignore actual dosing information tend to estimate biased clearance and volume and markedly overestimate random interindividual variability. Furthermore, data summarization strategies yield identical information but allow a large reduction in computer processing time, thus proving that simulation can be used for more efficient data analysis.

De Klerk and Urquhart[24] independently created a simpler Markov model based on two probabilities: one, observed from the patient's dosing history, is the probability that if a dose were taken yesterday, it would be taken today; the other, is that if the dose were forgotten yesterday, the probability of today's dose being taken is 0.5. The results showed a good approximation of the simulated dosing histories when compared with the original time histories of dosing, and a large gain in predictive value using these two simple probabilities compared with the prescribed number of doses as input variable.

Vrijens and Goetghebeur[9] started from a binary history of dosing, retaining individual dosing patterns but not exact timing. The model incorporated time-dependent effects of treatment, the dependence of a patient's current dosing on measured past dosing, the effect of the day of the week and the evolution of compliance over time during the study period, and allowed for interaction of these variables. They observed a strong association between compliance over the previous 6 days and the probability that today's dose will be taken as prescribed. Interestingly, the model estimated compliance in both study groups as equal. Their actual data showed a declining rate of compliance over time in both study groups, which indicates a higher-order effect not included in their model.

These three models all use probabilities derived from actual dosing histories to predict subsequent drug intake. All three have reasonably good predictive power—but which model is preferable would be evident only by running all three in a variety of experimental situations. The most important result to emerge from these three independent efforts is the finding that the best predictor of a patient's future compliance is their past compliance. It will be most interesting to test how this prediction holds up in circumstances where patients are switched from one drug to another with greater or fewer side-effects, more or less frequent dosing regimens, or different forms of educational/instructional programs—all the various factors that are often said to be important determinants of compliance.

Given the good predictability provided by each of these models, it is logical to hypothesize stability of drug intake over longer periods of time. In other words, if a patient proves to be a good complier it is likely that he or she will stay a good complier, and if he or she is a variable complier future compliance is also likely to be variable. So far, however, this is only an assumption and further work is needed.

Validation

Once a model has been devised, it is by no means finished. Like any scientific method, it must be validated against known information. The objective of validation is to create a model that is as good as the information available at that moment, and to stimulate experimental work to broaden the range of available data to challenge the model's ability to simulate with reasonable precision. A logical step with a presumably reliable model of patient compliance is to use its projections about future intake of drug as input to pharmacokinetic/pharmacodynamic models not only to project the history of drug concentration in plasma (as did Rubio et al.[23]) but also to project the time course of the drug's actions.

Here, however, we encounter a curious gap in our knowledge. There is abundant data showing the high incidence of sudden halts in dosing for variously long periods but the pharmacodynamic data available include very little information that would allow us to predict the time course of a drug's action (with or without rebound effects or recurrent first-dose effects) when dosing is suddenly but temporarily interrupted. In other words, the available pharmacodynamic models are insufficiently constrained because they function on the basis of an assumption, unsupported by data, on the time course of drug action when dosing halts. There would be no difficulty if we could rely on the assumption that a drug's action is predicted by the time course of its concentration in plasma but one need not look far to see how poor an assumption that is. The presently best-selling pharmaceutical, omeprazole, has a plasma half-life of 30–60 minutes[25] and a post-dose duration of action of 3–4 days[26]. There is an evident need for pharmacometricians to fill in the missing data by extending the sampling times in multidose phase I and II studies—and not to stop sampling when the last dose is given, but to continue until all manifestations of the drug's action have disappeared.

If the validation procedure satisfies the requirements of the model, it is possible to introduce variable compliance by varying the input, and to project the effect of variable compliance on the selected outcome parameters. The optimal way of representing variable compliance differs from situation to situation. One good way is to use the distribution of variable interdose-intervals that seem likely to pose compliance-related problems (as described above). Other possibilities to compare are hypothetical high-risk and low-risk patterns, or to use a distribution of all interdose-intervals possible. The outcomes projected by the model can be used to assess the loss of efficacy and the occurrence of safety problems (e.g. rebound or recurrent first-dose effects) and other compliance-related problems under varying conditions.

The simulation alone is not a sufficient answer. It is like running an unvalidated test, which may or may not be accurate; there is no way to be sure. However, a growing body of confirmed simulations increases the confidence in the ability of the model to project the consequences of unexplored situations. In any case, depending on the specific situation, the moment of development at which the simulation is done and the quality of the information in the model, it is possible to use the outcomes to anticipate specific problems. Examples are the use of a drug delivery system to extend duration of action and thus make the drug more 'forgiving' to variable interdose intervals, or labeling information to address special properties.

CONCLUSIONS

Electronic monitoring has given a great insight into the day-by-day variability of outpatient drug intake. The resulting variability in interdose intervals is not adequately addressed in current drug development. One way of doing so is to use computer-aided simulation to create a model to link drug intake (input) to drug actions (and side-effects) (outcomes). Validation of the model is an ongoing task, but confidence in the model grows as it satisfactorily simulates an increasingly diverse array of inputs. Once a model is created, it is possible to run several simulations of variable drug intake, which can mimic 'usual outpatient compliance', high-risk patterns, low-risk patterns, or a whole theoretical spectrum of drug intake patterns, with particular attention paid to outliers, in whom a combination of unlikely circumstances could cause serious harm. The results can be used to anticipate compliance-related problems, adapt delivery systems if necessary, or use in drug labeling or marketing.

Compliance simulation models can also be incorporated in trial simulation software, introducing variable drug intake as a real and prevalent source of bias, thereby anticipating problems that may be avoided by various means—better labeling, altered dose regimen, use of drug delivery technology, etc. Most importantly, however, these models show that drug development should take advantage of new methods of measuring drug exposure, thereby increasing the quality of drug development and hopefully providing physicians and patients with better therapeutics.

REFERENCES

1. Feinstein AR. On white-coat effects and the electronic monitoring of compliance. *Arch Intern Med* 1990; **150:** 1377–8
2. Bond WS, Hussar DA. Detection methods and strategies for improving medication compliance. *Am J Hosp Pharm* 1991; **48:** 1978–88
3. Cramer JA, Mattson RH, Prevey ML, Scheyer RD, Ouellette VL. How often is medication taken as prescribed? A novel assessment technique. *JAMA* 1989; **261:** 3273–7
4. Vander Stichele R. Measurement of patient compliance and the interpretation of randomized clinical trials. *Eur J Clin Pharmacol* 1991; **41:** 27–35
5. Kruse W, Weber E. Dynamics of drug regimen compliance—its assessment by microprocessor-based monitoring. *Eur J Clin Pharmacol* 1990; **38:** 561–5
6. de Klerk E. Patient compliance in hypertension. *CardioTopics* 1997; **1:** 7–21
7. Pullar T, Kumar S, Tindall H, Feely M. Time to stop counting the tablets? *Clin Pharmacol Ther* 1989; **46:** 163–8
8. Urquhart J. The electronic medication event monitor—lessons for pharmacotherapy. *Clin Pharmacokinet* 1997; **32:** 345–56
9. Vrijens B, Goetghebeur E. Comparing compliance patterns between randomized treatments. *Contr Clin Trials* 1997; **18:** 187–203
10. Girard P, Sheiner LB, Kastrissios H, Blaschke TF. Do we need full compliance data for population pharmacokinetic analysis? *J Pharmacokinet Biopharm* 1996; **24:** 265–81
11. de Klerk E, van der Linden SJ. Compliance monitoring of NSAID drug therapy in ankylosing spondylitis, experiences with an electronic monitoring device. *Br J Rheumatol* 1996; **35:** 60–5
12. Vander Stichele RH. Time intervals between medication events: an approach to measurement of patient compliance with data from electronic monitoring. Seminar, University of Limburg, Diepenbeek, Belgium, 1993.
13. Urquhart J, Chevalley C. Impact of unrecognized dosing errors on the cost and effectiveness of pharmaceuticals. *Drug Inform J* 1988; **22:** 363–78
14. The Lipid Research Clinics Coronary Primary Prevention Trial results. I. Reduction in incidence of coronary heart disease. *JAMA* 1984; **251:** 351–64
15. The Lipid Research Clinics Coronary Primary Prevention Trial results. II. The relationship of reduction in incidence of coronary heart disease to cholesterol lowering. *JAMA* 1984; **251:** 365–74
16. Johnson BF, Whelton A. A study design for comparing the effects of missing daily doses of antihypertensive drugs. *Am J Ther* 1994; **1:** 1–8

17. Vanhove GF, Schapiro JM, Winters MA, Merigan TC, Blaschke TF. Patient compliance and drug failure in protease inhibitor monotherapy [letter]. *JAMA* 1996; **276:** 1955–6

18. Rudd P. Compliance with antihypertensive therapy: a shifting paradigm. *Cardiol Rev* 1994; **2:** 230–40

19. Rudd P, Ahmed S, Zachary V, Barton C, Bonduelle D. Compliance with medication timing: implications from a medication trial for drug development and clinical practice. *J Clin Res Pharmacoepidemiol* 1992; **6:** 15–27

20. Kruse W, Nikolaus T, Rampmaier J, Weber E, Schlierf G. Actual versus prescribed timing of lovastatin doses assessed by electronic compliance monitoring. *Eur J Clin Pharmacol* 1993; **45:** 211–15

21. Waterhouse DM, Calzone KA, Mele C, Brenner DE. Adherence to oral tamoxifen: a comparison of patient self-report, pill counts, and microelectronic monitoring. *J Clin Oncol* 1993; **11:** 1189–97

22. de Klerk E, van der Linden S, van der Heijde D, Urquhart J. Facilitated analysis of data on drug regimen compliance. *Stat Med* 1997; **16:** 1653–64

23. Rubio A, Cox C, Weintraub M. Prediction of diltiazem plasma concentration curves from limited measurements using compliance data. *Clin Pharmacokinet* 1992; **22:** 238–46

24. de Klerk E. Range and Predictability of Drug Exposure in Clinical Trials: Electronic Monitoring. DIA conference: Drug Compliance Issues in Clinical Trials and Patient Care, European Workshop, Paris, 30.09–10.01 1996, 1996.

25. Goodman Gilman A, Rall TD, Nies AS, Taylor P. *The pharmacological basis of therapeutics.* 8th edition. New York: Pergamon Press, 1990: 902–4

26. Lind T, Cederberg C, Ekenved G, Hagland U, Olbe L. Effect of omeprazol—a gastric proton pump inhibitor—on pentagastrin stimulated acid secretion in man. *Gut* 1983; **24:** 270–6

5

Promises of a Measurement Breakthrough

Robert Vander Stichele

Heymans Institute of Pharmacology, University of Gent, Gent, Belgium

THE LONG AND WINDING ROAD OF COMPLIANCE RESEARCH

The medical community awakened to the problem of compliance in the mid-1970s, with a first major medical congress on the topic in 1975[1], and the publication of a widely read book[2]. Ever since there has been a stream of publications on the subject. However, what at first seemed an explosive growth in new emerging scientific discipline[3] soon turned into a stagnating field, without much bibliographic rigor[4] and without major scientific breakthroughs.

Peter Rudd in 1979 pinpointed the 'Achilles heel' of compliance research: the lack of a 'gold standard' in measurement[5]. Stressing the same point, Herbert Caron[6] concluded that 'the intelligence, energy and productivity of research groups was largely wasted, because of the failure to insist on objective quantification and experimental design'. Leventhal pointed out that the lack of a theoretical framework hinders our understanding of compliance and the development of measurements techniques[7]. In one of the latest critical reviews of the achievements of compliance research, Morris[8] concluded that 'after decades of compliance research, very little consistent information is available, except that people do not take their medications as prescribed.' Morris further pointed out that the field has focused on description of the extent of the phenomenon, on an unfruitful attempt to discover the determinants of non-compliance, without regard to a theoretical framework, lacking in conceptual rigor, hampered by methodological flaws and dominated by the perspective of the health professional[8].

A recent attempt to update the current knowledge on interventions to improve compliance was made in a systematic review in *The Lancet*[9]. An extensive literature search produced only 13 randomized clinical trials,

Drug Regimen Compliance: Issues in Clinical Trials and Patient Management.
Edited by J.-M. Métry and U.A. Meyer. © 1999 John Wiley & Sons Ltd.

selected after evaluating a limited set of quality criteria. Eight of these studies were underpowered. The interventions were a disparate collection of actions, undertaken in treatment of hypertension, neuropsychiatric disorders and acute infections. The average age of the studies was 13 years and the generalizability of the results was questionable. The validity of the methods of compliance measurement in these studies was not discussed in the review. None of the trials used the newer measurement methods (low dose markers—phenobarbital or digoxin—or electronic monitoring) and the author did not discuss the potential impact of these innovations. This omission is strange as the author himself called for a 'dramatic change and a serious research effort to deepen our understanding of compliance and our ability to improve patients' self-administration of prescribed medicines, still the most common form of therapy'[9].

The annual count of articles published in MEDLINE from 1975 to 1996 with the keyword 'patient compliance' (Figure 5.1) demonstrates the stagnation and increasingly derivative nature of scientific production in the field, including slow diffusion of old findings in the different specialties and endless repetitions of discussions about compliance and adherence.

ELECTRONIC MONITORING: AN UNNOTICED REVOLUTION IN MEASUREMENT OF COMPLIANCE

Minor progress in measurement techniques includes the development of better questionnaires, the use of markers (low-dose phenobarbital, low-dose

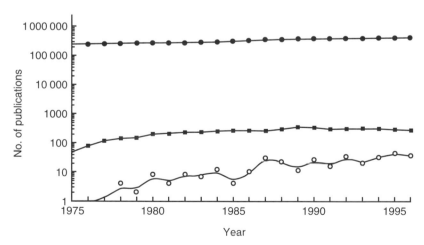

FIGURE 5.1 Stagnation in the annual production of patient compliance articles in MEDLINE, 1975–1996. ● Total number of articles published; ○ reviews containing the keywords 'patient compliance'; ■ articles containing the keywords 'patient compliance'

digoxin, deuterium oxide) and determination of active substances in hair. Institutionalized supervision of intake in AIDS patients is not a new measurement technique but a return to the draconian measures used to prevent the possibility of non-compliance in tuberculosis patients.

A true scientific revolution, in the Kuhnian sense of the term, is the advent of electronic monitoring of medication. The idea behind this is to fit an ordinary pill container with an electronic device to record the opening of the container. The device not only counts but also time-stamps the openings and collects this information into a downloadable memory. Hence, it is possible to review retrospectively the medication events of periods of therapy, from one week of acute treatment to several months of chronic therapy. This electronic recording of the acts of taking medication provides a unique method for time-stamping a repetitive human behaviour. The first expensive, bulky and fragile experimental devices have now evolved into affordable, practical and reliable measurement instruments.

Electronic monitoring is clearly a revolution, bringing a new era of precision to the field of compliance research. It provides the possibility of locating drug holidays within long periods of therapy and of linking these holidays to clinical events. The difference between dosing once, twice, three or four times a day can be studied on a daily basis over long periods of time. Temporal patterns in patient compliance can be followed, as patients pass from start-up therapy to routine sustainment of chronic therapy and eventually discontinuation. New composite measures of patient compliance can be produced, such as the percentage of days within a period of therapy with correct dosing, or the percentage of doses taken at the correct times. As the exact time of successive dosing events is known, the dosing interval (time between two dosing events) can be calculated and used as a unit of analysis. All this is much more relevant and valid than the inaccurate and imprecise measure provided by the pill count, until now the dominant measurement methodology in compliance research.

This innovation in compliance measurement has in fact been around for more than 20 years[10]. Electronic monitoring was pioneered with eyedrop dispensers by ophthalmologists[11,12], who must have been fascinated by their observances of poorly compliant glaucoma patients knowingly sliding into blindness from optic nerve damage in relatively short lapses of time. Ten years later, several experimental and commercial devices were developed for oral medications[13-15]. By 1988, the clinical implications of this new measurement technique had been fully discussed[16] and electronic monitoring was included in a methodological review of compliance measurement methods[17]. The current state of this research field has been recently reviewed[18,19].

However, electronic monitoring has only been slowly adopted and by a minority in the research community: reviews on patient compliance continue to be written and published without mentioning this new method. Pharmaceutical companies, clinical investigators and scholars in compliance have failed to distinguish a major scientific breakthrough from a gadget and continue to plan and conduct volunteer phase 1 studies, clinical efficacy trials and compliance studies without using electronic monitoring, and even without explaining why electronic monitoring was not used.

FOCUSING ON MODIFYING COMPLIANCE BY THE PROVISION OF PATIENT INFORMATION

In this chapter we will illustrate the impact of the methodological breakthrough in compliance measurement on the research strategies within a small (well delimited) research field. It is a testimony from our experience with research into the effects of patient package inserts (PPIs) on patient behavior.

The PPI is a piece of paper stuffed inside medication boxes, designed to be read by the patient shortly after he or she buys medication from the pharmacist, whether or not on prescription. The insert may or may not be read a second time, depending on whether in the course of therapy problems arise that are perceived as drug-related.

The pharmaceutical industry is pioneering a marketing concept in which the product, the brand name and the written information that goes with it form an unbreakable unit at the point of sale. The insert is not just a manual for use but a vehicle for relevant information on the risks of the medicine, so that the consumer is fully informed on the benefits and risks of the proposed therapy.

Since 1992 legislation has mandated the inclusion of understandable inserts containing full information in the package of every branded medicine sold in any of the countries of the European Community. In the USA, the FDA advocates a similar approach in its MEDGUIDE proposal. FDA approval is pending for a waiting period where the private sector (industry, pharmacists and physicians) is challenged to assure sufficient distribution of information at the point of sale of drugs in a voluntary way. If, after a waiting period, the private sector has not reached its targets, this proposal will come into force. These legislative initiatives have been driven by the desire to fulfill the 'right to know' of the consumer. However, in the often fierce debates about the sense or non-sense of this approach, both positive and negative aspects of the written information on patient compliance have been postulated.

It is clear that improving patient compliance is not a trivial matter and that complex interventions are needed to achieve a positive effect on adherence as well as on outcome. It is highly unlikely that a weak intervention such as the provision of written information will achieve spectacular effects. However, improving patient compliance is not the only target of the provision of inserts: intense study of other variables (the number of people who read the information, patient satisfaction and knowledge of the medication) has clearly shown that explicit and clear information has positive effects[20]. Moreover, the PPI can induce a more intense perception of a medication's risks and benefits[21].

The impact of the PPI on compliance has been examined in many studies, but mostly using poor measurement tools, producing rather unconvincing and sometimes conflicting results[22]. Because of these disappointing results, there was a gradual and insidious shift in the primary objective of the patient information programs in the 1990s, from the assurance of patient compliance towards the assurance of adequate reactions of patients in case of side-effects and overdosing, which have been clearly linked to hospital admissions[23]. In the rationale and in the cost–benefit analysis of the MEDGUIDE program, the FDA clearly points towards the possibility of reducing the staggering cost of drug-related hospital admission as the primary motive for engaging in a mandatory drug information provision program[24]. There are some opportunities in Europe to test the hypothesis that, on a macroeconomic scale, the impact of written PPIs should be observable by studying the difference in rate of drug-related hospital admissions between countries with and without PPIs in their drug distribution system, and in countries shifting from drug distribution without written information towards a system using PPIs. Continuous monitoring of drug-related hospital admissions was proposed as a quality indicator of ambulatory care in general and of informational status of patients in particular[25].

Research now should concentrate on how to clearly communicate the 'risk' messages without jeopardizing compliance[26]. There may be some sense in building messages into the PPI to support the compliance enhancing efforts of care givers and health professionals, but it is probably an illusion to believe that this piece of paper will enhance, on its own, patient compliance.

Multiple combinations of interventions to improve patient compliance are possible, such as intensive training of physicians to change the physician–patient interaction, counseling of patients by nurses and pharmacists and public information campaigns[27,28]. The provision of written drug information on a massive scale within the drug distribution process is just one intervention and should be part of a complex mixture of interventions. To optimize the impact of patient package inserts, we need a clear understanding on how to write the best possible insert, and how to best fit it into the context of provision of information, caring for patients and ensuring patient compliance to prescribed therapy.

The question is now: 'how will we research ways to design PPIs that will achieve the desired outcomes of readership, satisfaction, knowledge, correct risk/benefit perception and adequate reactions to adverse events without endangering compliance?' While trying to answer that question we will highlight the role of electronic monitoring.

METHODOLOGICAL APPROACHES OF EVALUATING THE IMPACT OF PATIENT INFORMATION ON COMPLIANCE

Research in this field will be fruitful only when it results from an elaborated theoretical model, when it tests well written patient information, when it employs innovative study designs and when it applies new, precise measurement tools for relevant intermediate variables, for patient compliance and, last but not least, outcome. Only a combination of these items will enable us to detect the clues for designing better PPIs, to maximize the small benefits they induce and to avoid unwanted effects. This complicated quest for little changes is important because of the massive scale on which these inserts are deployed once they become part of the drug distribution process.

In this chapter we discuss a long-lasting research program which evaluated the shift from technical inserts to patient package inserts during the period 1988–1992 in the drug distribution system of Belgium.

Theoretical Framework

This research program started from the assumption that the results of an intervention study regarding patient compliance are limited to the clinical setting of the study, which is determined by the characteristics of the disease (acute/chronic, symptomatic/asymptomatic, curable/alleviable) and the characteristics of the treatment (accompanied by frequent minor side-effects or not, associated with serious risk or not, vulnerable to non-compliance or not). The characteristics of disease and treatment are intricately related and can hardly be studied separately. Therefore, we proposed the term 'drug–disease dyad', to accurately describe and categorize clinical settings. Examples include curable cancer–hair-loss-inducing oncologic treatment; hypertension–beta-blockers; acute bronchitis–antibiotics; AIDS–experimental treatment; tuberculosis–streptomycin; epilepsy–carbamazepine; asthma–inhaled steroids.

On the one hand we acknowledge the diversity of clinical situations but on the other we need a common classification of different types of non-compliance. In the review a categorical classification into six types of compliance, based on alterations of the risk–benefit ratio, was proposed (Table 5.1)[29].

TABLE 5.1 Risk–benefit classification of non-compliance for a prescribed drug regimen

	Risk	Benefit
Complier	Acceptable	Optimal
Partial complier	Strong	Suboptimal
Overuser	Strong	(Sub)optimal
Erratic user	Strong	Doubtful
Partial dropout	Moderate	—
Dropout*	—	—

*Dropout is not part of the classic definition of non-compliance

For each drug–disease dyad, relevant classes and demarcation criteria should be used to assign patients with a specific behavior to each class. For example, for asthma all six classes are needed, while for hypertension the distinction between complier, partial complier and dropout may suffice. Determining the impact of partial compliance (occasional omission of doses within otherwise regular therapy) must be carefully assessed. The pharmacokinetic and pharmacodynamic properties of the drug, and hence the duration of action of the drug, must be taken into consideration.

Only electronic monitoring provides enough information on the different aspects of non-compliance to discriminate between behaviors. Researchers will need to define *a priori* in the protocol the demarcation criteria to use when classifying patients on the basis of compliance monitoring data.

In our studies we used a number of background theories to guide the elaboration of experiments. We worked with Ley's cognitive model[30], because it provided a schema to combine the role of information and the role of emotions such as satisfaction and fear in the compliance behavior. We worked with the more heuristic approach of Paul Slovic to study risk perception and a lay person's judgment in uncertainty[31] and adopted the cognitive psychology theory of self-efficacy[32] to study behavioral changes provoked by information and the occurrence of side-effects.

We concentrated on three different instances of compliance in relation to the onset and halting of therapy:

1. The coping decision to accept the prescription and start taking the medicine.
2. The coping decision to continue treatment as a routine procedure and, whenever clinically meaningful events occur (such as worsening of the disease, dissipation of the symptoms of the disease, presence of side-effects).
3. Discontinuation or compliance deteriorating with time, due to lack of motivation.

Electronic monitoring makes it feasible to study these three phases of therapy, either separately or in a continuous time frame.

A small experimental study[33] led us to the hypothesis that written drug information enhances the attribution of body symptoms (side-effects or not) to the medication taken. Some medicines cause body symptoms in most patients, either by fluctuating attenuation of disease symptoms, or by dose-related 'minor' side-effects. It is possible that this provokes greater irregularity of timing, more drug holidays and, hence, lesser patient compliance. The effect could be worsened by explicit written information, certainly if the patient is not warned by the healthcare provider to anticipate problems. The precision of electronic monitoring is necessary to pick up these small differences with sufficient power in studies with a reasonable sample size.

An experimental study in the clinical setting of alleviating treatment of acute locomotor trauma using NSAIDs[21] indicated the capability of clear, explicit information to alter patients' risk/benefit perception and their readiness to report side-effects.

We have created a qualitative model to study the impact of written drug information on patient compliance, integrating the elements mentioned above (Figure 5.2). This model must be further tested empirically.

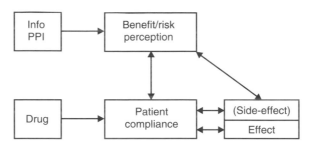

FIGURE 5.2 Model for the study of the impact of written drug information, presented as a patient package insert, on risk/benefit perception and patient compliance as intermediate variables in the causal relationship between drug and drug effects and/or side-effects

Powerful Intervention Tools

Readability is an obvious prerequisite for written patient information to be effective. However, readability should be tested by objective criteria. We developed a computerized readability testing program (for the Dutch and the French languages), based on classics such as word length, sentence length and basic terminology, and augmented with more elaborate testing of grammatical complexity and, above all, the occurrence of context-specific medical jargon[25].

The more readable a text is, the more naked the information it conveys. Writing a good patient package insert is not only a linguistic problem but also a question of communicative quality. The writer should have a clear communication strategy, guided by explicit objectives and a rich theoretical model.

An early study of the motives of patients to read the insert[34] had taught us to categorize the many messages inside a patient package insert into three different areas (procedural information, risk information and background information). This categorization proved useful in writing high-quality PPIs and hence in producing powerful intervention tools.

In a classical insert, the risk information dominates and messages on the benefits of the medicine are often absent (usually they have been banned by the regulatory authorities because of fear of advertising in a document with public status). There is very little research on the potential impact of information on benefit in the insert. Recent experimental studies indicate that objectively formulated benefit messages strongly influence patient perception. However, this needs to be tested further in clinical studies where electronic monitoring is used to detect subtle group differences.

Measurement Tools

Methodological research is needed to aid development of valid and precise scales of the perception of benefit and risk of medication in the clinical setting. We need tools to measure relevant emotions such as fear and satisfaction at crucial intervals in the cascade of patient–physician–drug-information interaction. We need questionnaires that will probe patients for the occurrence of specific common side-effects and body symptoms and ask them whether they attribute these symptoms to their drug[21]. This results in the reporting of higher percentages of side-effects than with more traditional systems of passive reception of side-effects reported by the patient. It takes some courage for pharmaceutical companies to conduct this kind of research and to allow publication of results that are easily drawn out of context and misrepresented by competitors.

Of course, a highly sensitive and accurate measurement tool is needed for the key variable of patient compliance. The lack of such a tool has hampered the efforts of the field for many years. Electronic monitoring makes it possible to relate dosing events to the timing of informational interventions and the occurrence of side-effects. To pick up small effects, it might be necessary to study compliance with the dosing interval (the time between a dose and the next dose) as the unit of analysis.

Statistical Issues

More precise measurement will strengthen statistical analysis. The possibility of observing and measuring a more diverse array of aspects of non-compliance (e.g. dosing accuracy, timing accuracy, temporal aspects) will enable the researcher to classify patients reliably into strictly delimited categories (e.g. punctual compliers, partial compliers and non-compliers). This will, in turn, enable powerful subgroup analysis of the punctual compliers. New statistical approaches to that end are under development[34].

Design Issues

Electronic monitoring turns any clinical trial into a naturalistic study of dosing omissions. Using this methodology it is possible to study the natural experiments in which patients engage when they skip therapy for one (or a few more) days and to correlate these omissions to clinical events.

It is also possible to design studies where active substances are given for longer periods, and (at prespecified days) replaced for one or more days by placebo, in a double-blinded way. Electronic monitoring can then record changes in drug taking behavior induced by the weaning of pharmacological action of the substance under study.

As well as experiments in clinical psychology, there is a need for randomized clinical trials within the natural care setting, such as in general practice. This is an exciting but difficult endeavor. Although methodologically preferable, it will be difficult (and sometimes ethically impossible) to conduct placebo-controlled trials to test hypotheses on the impact of information. In such studies, the comparator is more likely to be an active ingredient. It is difficult to reconcile the demand of concealment of allocation in a double-blind randomized controlled trial with the need to test the impact of information on two active compounds. Each of the two medicines to be tested has a different set of side-effects. Providing a PPI with the matching information would break the blinding for the physician and ultimately also for the patient. Therefore a hybrid text must be created containing relevant information from both medicines (Figure 5.3). Blinded medicine is thus provided with an identical text in both arms of the trial. This approach solves the dilemma between blinding and correct information.

The Broader Context

Finally, the context of providing written drug information should be more thoroughly studied. We conducted a survey to explore the attitude of prescribing physicians to written drug information[35]. The results indicate that a serious educational effort is needed to persuade physicians of the value of written drug information and of a positive interaction with this medium.

Pharmacists appear much more proactively involved in research to optimize pharmaceutical care through counseling and provision of information. In some studies, electronic monitoring is not just used as a measurement device: the information it provides (a detailed history of individual drug-taking behavior) is used as a feedback intervention to the patient.

CONCLUSION

The advent of electronic monitoring of patient compliance means that scientific research now stands a chance of producing a solid theoretical framework and practical clinical remedies for the widespread problem of noncompliance. Well written patient package inserts will play a modest but crucial role in modern drug distribution systems for ambulatory care.

WHAT THE MEDICINE IS FOR

Your doctor has prescribed this medicine in a clinical study of high blood pressure treatment (hypertension). This medicine lowers blood pressure to the normal level. High blood pressure damages blood vessels, the heart, the brain, and the kidneys. This may lead to a heart attack, a stroke, or kidney failure. Taking the medicine lowers the risk of these events.

HOW TO TAKE, HOW MUCH TO TAKE

Take one tablet each day, in the morning. You can take the tablet before, during, after or without breakfast.

WHO SHOULD NOT TAKE THIS MEDICINE

You should NOT take this medicine if:
> you have severe trouble with heart rhythm
> > (second or third degree block);
> you are under 14 years of age;
> you have a severe kidney disease;
> you are taking the drug called verapamil
> > (Fibrocard®, Isoptine®, Lodixal®);
> you are allergic to any component of this medicine;
> you are pregnant, planning pregnancy, or nursing.

SIDE-EFFECTS

The following side-effects sometimes occur: dizzy spells, headache, tiredness or fatigue, nausea, diarrhea, cold feet, muscle weakness, or slowing of the heart beat. Some patients may develop a persistent cough. Less frequently, patients may have difficulty sleeping. Any of these side-effects should be discussed with the doctor at the next visit.

Exceptionally, patients may develop a skin rash or have difficulty breathing or feel a swelling of the face, lips, tongue, or throat. In that case, patients should promptly consult their doctor. These signs may signal that an allergy to the medicine has developed.

SPECIAL PRECAUTIONS

Patients who recently followed a low salt diet, patients who suffered from vomiting or diarrhea should inform their doctor. Patients with asthma, heart failure, problems with heart rhythm, or kidney disease should also inform their doctor. They may need to be seen more regularly.

It is hazardous to suddenly stop this medicine. Do not stop the medicine without first consulting your doctor. Your doctor will tell you how to step safely out of the treatment.

Be sure to mention that you take this medicine, in case you need to be put to sleep for surgery.

PREGNANCY AND NURSING

If you are pregnant or want to become pregnant, you must inform your doctor. Pregnant or nursing women should not take this medicine.

DRIVING VEHICLES AND OPERATING MACHINERY

This medicine does not pose any special hazards for driving or operating machinery.

WHAT TO DO IN CASE OF AN OVERDOSE

Overdoses cause a drop of the blood pressure and drop of the heart rate to dangerously low levels. Patients with overdoses need hospital care.

OTHER MEDICINES

Tell your doctor about all the medicines that you are taking. Patients should inform their doctor, when they are taking the drug called clonidine (Catapressan®, Dixarit®).

PACKAGING

Sixty tablets are packaged in a round bottle.

STORING THE MEDICINE

Store the medicine in a cool, dry place. Refrigeration is not necessary. Avoid direct contact with sunlight.

FIGURE 5.3 Hybrid patient package insert for a randomized controlled trial involving atenolol and lisinopril

REFERENCES

1. Haynes RB, Taylor DW, Sackett DL. *Compliance in health care.* Johns Hopkins University Press, Baltimore, 1979.
2. Lasagna L. *Patient compliance.* Futura, Mount Kisco (NY), 1976.
3. Lüscher TF, Vetter H, Siegnehaler W, Wetter W. Compliance in hypertension: facts and concepts. *J Hypertens* 1985;**3**[suppl 1]:3–9.
4. Bauer JT. Methodological rigor and citation frequency in patient compliance literature. *Am J Public Health* 1982;**72**:9–23.
5. Rudd P. In search for the gold standard for compliance measurement [editorial]. *Arch Intern Med* 1979;**139**:627–8.
6. Caron HS. Compliance: the case for objective measurement. *J Hypertens* 1985;**3**[suppl 1]:11–17.
7. Leventhal H. The role of theory in the study of adherence to treatment and doctor–patient interactions. *Med Care* 1985;**23**:556–63.
8. Morris LS. Patient compliance: an overview. *J Clin Pharm Ther* 1992;**17**:283–95.
9. Haynes RB, McKibbon KA, Kanani R. Systematic review of randomized trials of interventions to assist patients to follow prescriptions for medications. *Lancet* 1996;**348**:383–86.
10. Kass MA, Zimmerman T, Yablonski M, Becker B. Compliance to pilocarpine therapy. *Invest Ophthalmol* 1977;**108**: Abstract 2.
11. Norrell SE, Granstrom PA, Wassen R. A medication monitor and fluorescein technique designed to study medication behaviour. *Acta Ophthalmol* 1980;**58**:459–67.
12. Kass MA, Gordon M, Meltzer DW. Can ophthalmologists correctly identify patients defaulting from pilocarpine therapy? *Am J Ophthalmol* 1986;**101**:524–30.
13. Eisen SA, Hanpeter JA, Kreuger LW, Gard M. Monitoring medication compliance: descriptions of a new device. *J Compliance Health Care* 1987;**2**:131–42.
14. Cheung R, Dickins J, Nicholson PW, Thomas ASC, Smith HH, Larson HE, Deshmukh AA, Dobbs RJ, Dobbs SM. Compliance with anti-tuberculous therapy: a field trial of a pill-box with a concealed recording device. *Eur J Clin Pharmacol* 1988;**35**:401–7.
15. Averbuch M, Weintraub M, Pollock DJ. Compliance in clinical trials: the MEMS device. *Clin Pharmacol Ther* 1988;**43**:185.
16. Urquhart J, Chevalley C. Impact of unrecognized dosing errors on the cost and the effectiveness of pharmaceuticals. *Drug Inform J* 1988;**22**:363–78.
17. Vander Stichele R. Measurement of patient compliance and the interpretation of randomized clinical trials. *Eur J Clin Pharmacol* 1991;**41**:27–35.
18. Urquhart J. The electronic medication event monitor—lessons for pharmacotherapy. *Clin Pharmacokinet* 1997;**32**:345–56.
19. Kastrissios H, Blaschke TF. Medication compliance as a feature in drug development. *Ann Rev Pharmacol Toxicol* 1997;**37**:451–75.
20. Vander Stichele RH, Bogaert MG. European legislation and research projects regarding patient education for medication. *Drug Inform J* 1995;**29**:285–90.
21. Vanhaecht CHM, Vander Stichele R, De Backer G, Bogaert MG. Impact of patient package inserts on patients' satisfaction, adverse drug reactions and risk perception: the case of NSAIDs for posttraumatic pain relief. *Pat Educ Counsel* 1991;**17**:205–15.
22. Mullen PD, Green LW, Persinger GS. Clinical trials of patient education for chronic conditions: a comparative meta-analysis of intervention types. *Prev Med* 1985;**14**:735–81.

23. Wagdi P, Vuilliomenet A, Kaufmann U, Richter M, Bertel O. Inadequate treatment compliance, patient information and drug prescriptions as causes for emergency hospitalisation of patients with chronic heart failure [German]. *Schweiz Med Wochenschr* 1993;**123**:108–12.

24. FDA. Prescription drug product labeling; Medication guide requirements. Proposed rule. *Fed Reg* 1995;**60**:44182–252.

25. Vander Stichele R. Side effects of medicines and partial compliance: two related impediments to the quality of prescription drug therapy. *Abstracts of the 31 Annual meeting of the Drug Information Association*, 1995, p. 145.

26. Morris LA. *Communicating therapeutic risks*. Springer Verlag, New York, 1990.

27. DiMatteo MR. Enhancing patient adherence in medical recommendations. *JAMA* 1994;**271**:79–83.

28. De Geest S. *Subclinical noncompliance with cyclosporine therapy in heart transplant recipients. A cluster analytic study*. Doctoral Thesis. University of Leuven, 1996.

29. Vander Stichele RH, Vanhaecht CH, Braem MD, Bogaert MG. Attitude of the public towards technical package inserts for medication information in Belgium. *DICP* 1991;**25**:1002–6.

30. Ley P, Morris L. The psychology of written information for patients. In: Rachman S, ed. *Contributions to medical psychology*. New York, Pergamon Press, 1994.

31. Slovic P. Kraus NN, Lappe H, Letzel H, Malfors T. Risk perception of prescription drugs: report of a survey in Sweden. In: Horisberger B, Dinkel R, eds. *The perception and management of drug safety risks*. New York, Springer Verlag, 1989.

32. Leventhal H, Safer MA, Panagis DM. The impact of communications on the self regulation of health beliefs, decisions and behavior. *Health Educ Q* 1983;**10**:3–29.

33. Vander Stichele RH, Thomson M, Verkoelen K, Droussin AM. Measuring patient compliance with electronic monitoring: lisinopril versus atenolol in essential hypertension. *Post Marketing Surveillance* 1992;**6**:77–90.

34. Goetghebeur EJT, Pocock SJ. Statistical issues in allowing for noncompliance and withdrawal. *Drug Inform J* 1993;**27**:837 15.

35. Vander Stichele RH, De Potter B, Vyncke P, Bogaert MG. Attitude of physicians towards patient package inserts for medication information in Belgium. *Pat Educ Couns* 1996;**28**:5–13.

6

The Place of Microelectronic Systems in Measuring Compliance

Marie-Paule Schneider, Claire-Lise Fallab Stubi, Bernard Waeber and Michel Burnier

Policlinique Médicale Universitaire and Division d'Hypertension et de Médecine Vasculaire, Lausanne, Switzerland

INTRODUCTION

Patient compliance, which can be defined as the extent to which a person's behavior coincides with health-related advice, has long been recognized as an important clinical problem[1,2]. Indeed, all practitioners know very well that their patients do not routinely follow their instructions and numerous studies conducted using directed interviews, questionnaires, pill counts or blood and urine tests have demonstrated that adherence to drug therapy is relatively poor (about 50%), regardless of the disease and the therapeutic regimen[3,4]. These studies have not only revealed the clinical relevance of non-compliance but have also enabled characterization of the various patterns of compliance (very regular, partial or totally erratic). Few patients appear to be over-compliant to prescribed regimens.

Until recently, precise clinical evaluation of drug compliance was relatively complex and therefore limited to clinical studies. Moreover, no single method was entirely satisfactory and none could be used as a 'gold standard'. New approaches to measurement of drug compliance have been developed using microelectronic monitoring systems[5-8]. One of these devices is the Medication Event Monitoring System (MEMS), produced by the Aprex Corporation, Fremont, California, USA. This container, which can contain pill and capsule medication formulations, is fitted with a special cap containing a microprocessor that records each opening of the cap as a presumptive dose[7]. The MEMS device has been used extensively in large phase II and phase III clinical trials in which it is essential to assess the efficacy of new therapeutic agents by taking compliance into consideration and by drawing the relation curve between the medication really taken and the clinical outcome. The

Drug Regimen Compliance: Issues in Clinical Trials and Patient Management.
Edited by J.-M. Métry and U.A. Meyer. © 1999 John Wiley & Sons Ltd.

MEMS system, which offers the unique opportunity to collect dynamic data on compliance, has also been used in smaller groups of patients to characterize the patterns and the frequency of non-compliance[7,9–16]. The results obtained with the MEMS have largely confirmed those gathered with earlier methods.

Even though non-compliance has been thoroughly documented and clearly defined, little progress has been made on the ways to improve adherence, and only few physicians apply the basic recommendations for compliance support. The purpose of this chapter is to discuss the potential benefits expected from the use of electronic monitoring systems in clinical practice. In our opinion, these new monitors could completely change compliance-related practices and greatly improve patient adherence to the management of their disease.

DETECTION: THE FIRST STEP IN IMPROVING COMPLIANCE

The detection of non-compliance is not always an easy task for the clinician. Some subjects are rapidly recognized as totally non-compliant because they never attend their appointments and/or do not renew their drug prescriptions; in these cases, the therapeutic end-points are generally not achieved and it is not rare that the patient admits his or her difficulties after a short discussion. In this context, the patient often admits that he or she is unconvinced of the importance of treatment. The detection of partial non-compliers is more problematic because such patients agree to be treated and intend to comply. There are several causes for intermittent non-compliance: forgetfulness, changes in schedule, presence of side-effects or variations in priorities[12,17,18]. Some factors, such as the occurrence of side-effects, are easy to detect; others, however, are more difficult to reveal and the patients themselves are not always conscious of occasionally forgetting to take their treatment. In clinical practice, these inadequate partial compliers (30–40% of the treated population) certainly represent the ideal target for intervention because they understand the need for treatment and are willing to improve.

So far, the recognition of compliance errors in clinical practice has been very rudimentary and frequently limited to one or two direct questions to the patient with a brief, non-judgemental discussion. In the absence of factual objective data to discuss, the patient–physician dialogue is based mainly on a confidence relationship and the physician fears to disrupt the patient's trust with apparently indiscreet questions which he never learned to ask. This may explain why, in our experience, physicians have more difficulties in starting a discussion on compliance problems than the patients themselves. In contrast, physicians have no difficulty in discussing other very serious clinical and ethical problems regarding the patient's life and death. Occasionally, plasma or urinary drug levels can be obtained at the consultation, but the value of these results is limited by the fact that they represent only one time point in the patient's history. Furthermore, because patients tend to take their drugs a few days before the clinical visit this type of drug monitoring often overestimates the level of compliance.

To improve the detection of patients with non-compliance problems, several demographic and disease factors have been identified as potential indicators or risk factors for non-compliance (Table 6.1)[17,18]. Major factors negatively affecting long-term compliance appear to be the number of daily doses, the number of medications to be taken, the occurrence and severity of side-effects and compatibility with the patient's daily activities. Factors such as

TABLE 6.1   Potential risk factors for non-compliance

Demographic:
    Age
    Gender
    Educational achievement
    Socioeconomic status
    Employment
    Ethnicity

Drug- and treatment-related:
    Number of doses per day
    Number of drugs to be taken (complexity of the treatment)
    Size and taste of the tablets
    Side-effects
    Packaging
    Treatment duration
    Cost of medications
    Compatibility of the dose regimen with daily activities

Disease-related:
    Type and duration of the disease
    Patient understanding of the disease
    Threat posed by the disease
    Presence or absence of symptoms
    Influence of the disease on the ability to cooperate (mental disorders)

Patient-related:
    Understanding of the disease and its consequences
    Perception of the threat posed by the disease
    Acceptance of the disease
    Comprehension of the cost benefit of the treatment
    Motivation of patient and family
    Possible support of family or neighbourhood

Patient–healthcare professional relationships:
    Circumstances surrounding the patient's visit (easy access to physician or health care)
    Quality and effectiveness of the interaction
    Time spent by the healthcare providers
    Attitude of the physician towards the patient's illness and treatment
    Involvement of the patient in decisions
    Quality of the communication and adequacy of the information provided

the patient's knowledge of the disease and treatment, the strength of the patient–physician relationship, the patient's psychological state and access to the physician have only a modest influence on long-term drug adherence. Other parameters (such as age, gender, educational achievement, ethnicity and socioeconomic status) seem to have little, if any, impact on compliance. These risk factors for non-compliance may sometimes be clinically useful; however, one must consider that an apparently insignificant factor may suddenly become an important cause of non-compliance and, conversely, a presumed indicator of poor compliance such as advanced age may be irrelevant, for example because the patient's relationship to family members or neighbours ensures adequate adherence. Thus, it is clear that the detection of non-compliance remains rather insufficient and imprecise in today's clinical practice and that there is a need for new, innovative methods.

A PLACE FOR ELECTRONIC MONITORS?

As mentioned previously, electronic monitoring systems have been used mainly by researchers doing clinical studies on new drugs and in selected practice situations where they confirmed the frequency and relevance of the non-compliance problem[9–16]. So far, these devices have rarely been applied to conventional clinical practice in order to improve the efficiency of care and substantially enhance the clinical benefits of therapy. Yet, electronic monitoring could detect compliance problems in ambulatory medicine and help patients follow prescriptions for medications: indeed, electronic monitoring is simple, easy to handle and relatively cheap if one takes into account the price of drugs and potential savings[15]. The reading of the data takes only a few minutes. In contrast to blood and urine samples, which are sometimes considered as the gold standard, only electronic monitoring provides dynamic data regarding time and date of container opening. This aspect is crucial because compliance is by definition a dynamic parameter, which varies according to the patient's life. The compliance report that can be printed out from the collected data is another important aspect of the monitoring. The dose frequency is displayed as a calender plot indicating the number of openings occuring each day. This calender plot is very simple for the patient to understand and represents an interesting support enabling the physician to start a discussion with the patient based on real data rather than on suspicion. It is, of course, mandatory to inform the patient before starting monitoring and the main goal of the procedure must be to support rather than control drug compliance. This should enhance the patient's responsibility. The patient may feel very much concerned by the data that he or she has generated. With the compliance report in hand, it will be possible to involve the patient in devising solutions to correct the omissions during an interactive feedback discussion.

It may be argued that monitoring of drug compliance *per se* will probably improve adherence to treatment (the so-called 'study bias') but this apparent limitation may be turned into a potential advantage. The study bias can easily be used to demonstrate that the therapeutic goals can be reached—or not—if the treatment is taken correctly. Thus, depending on the degree of compliance measured and on the achievement of the treatment target (Table 6.2), the physician will be able to decide whether the patient needs a change in therapeutic regimen, additional information on drugs, compliance support or new investigations[19]. This type of approach could be particularly useful when dealing with patients who seem to be resistant to treatment. Indeed, it is crucial in this situation to distinguish non-compliance from therapeutic or diagnostic problems. The early recognition of non-adherence could save unnecessary and expensive investigations and prevent inappropriate changes in drug therapy.

So far, few investigators have taken advantage of the electronic monitoring system in clinical practice. To evaluate the usefulness of an electronic monitoring system in ambulatory medicine, we have recently used electronic monitoring in 30 asymptomatic patients receiving a chemoprophylaxis of isoniazide (300 mg/day) for 6 months[20]. The patients were seen monthly and electronic monitoring data were analysed at each visit by a pharmacist. Both the physician and the pharmacist discussed the calendar plots with the patient whenever necessary. As expected from the study bias, the overall mean compliance was greater than 90% in this study (91.5%), much higher than most reported data on compliance in the chemoprophylaxis of tuberculosis. More importantly, the use of electronic monitoring has enabled early detection of serious problems of non-compliance in four patients. With three, adequate overall compliance has finally been obtained by repeating the goals of therapy and discussing the data and the importance of the treatment. The fourth patient's compliance remains low, despite the various interventions. Electronic monitoring was well accepted by patients and physicians, the latter admitting that it is an interesting tool for recognizing and discussing compliance problems. In accordance with previous observations[6,10,15,16], we have found that both pill counting and a urine test for isoniazide overestimated

TABLE 6.2 Possible relationships between compliance results and therapeutic achievements

Compliance	Therapeutic goal	
	Achieved	Not achieved
>80%	Ideal. Educative value of compliance monitoring	Adapt treatment or consider diagnosis (investigations)
<80%	Re-evaluate diagnosis or reduce therapy	Re-emphasize the importance of compliance, propose compliance support

drug compliance, suggesting once more that electronic monitoring is the best way of assessing drug compliance in clinical practice.

ELECTRONIC MONITORING: THE ROLE OF THE PHARMACIST

Pharmacists could play a major role in the assessment and improvement of patient compliance; a role that has been recognized recently by the American Pharmaceutical Association, which has included in its specifications for new outpatient pharmacy services the identification of non-compliance, patient education and training and compliance monitoring[21].

In many European countries as well as in the USA, the pharmacist is responsible for the delivery of drugs and must provide counseling with every prescription dispensed. Providing information about medicines is certainly the most basic element of compliance promotion—a patient cannot take their drugs correctly if they do not know how. The pharmacist can very effectively recall the physician's instructions and supplement information as needed by the patient[13,21-24]. Multiple sources of information will help to prevent the patient forgetting and not understanding information provided by the various health professionals. The pharmacist can speak directly about compliance, promoting it by explaining the benefits of following treatment and the potential adverse effects of non-compliance. By doing so, he or she will help to increase the patient's education, a behavioral approach which has long been considered as the dominant method of improving patient compliance. Today, however, it is well recognized that education alone is better than no intervention but is insufficient to increase compliance[25].

It is as important for the pharmacist as for the physician to obtain feedback from the patient about his or her experiences and to assess compliance over time. Today, the pharmacy records represent the only accessible, verifiable estimates of compliance for use as feedback in a pharmacy[26]. An electronic monitoring system could be another method whereby the pharmacist can monitor drug adherence and improve compliance[13]. There are several reasons for involving the pharmacist in the monitoring process.

1. The prescribed drugs must be packed into the electronic device by a professional. If several drugs are to be monitored, it is essential to package them into different containers that can be differentiated by color. The patient instructions must be provided and the drug regimen indicated on the pill container.
2. It is crucial to explain precisely the functioning of the device and to remind the patient that he or she is free to accept or to refuse analysis of the data. It is not uncommon for a patient to accept the physician's proposal but to refuse monitoring when the device is presented by the pharmacist.

3. The pharmacist can discuss the patient's experience when they return for refills and help them to resolve any problems inhibiting proper medicine use. In this respect, he or she could propose specific aids such as refill reminder services. Patients are more likely to discuss the side-effects of their treatments with their pharmacist or with a practice nurse than their doctor[27].

In our opinion, electronic monitoring of drug compliance in ambulatory medicine should be performed in the context of a healthcare network involving the physician, the pharmacist and the patient. If necessary, visiting nurses and family members may also be involved in the network[23]. To evaluate the feasibility and the usefulness of a physician–pharmacist network for monitoring of drug compliance, a preliminary study has been carried out in which six pharmacies were completely equipped with the electronic monitoring system. Pharmacists were asked to contact their local physicians and to propose monitoring of drug compliance as a pharmacy service provided on the basis of a physician's prescription. The results of the assessments were analyzed by the pharmacist and addressed to the physician. Both healthcare providers discussed the collected data with their patients in order to improve compliance and to achieve the therapeutic goals. During the 6 months of the study, 133 physicians were contacted and 27 included patients, 37 of whom have received one or several electronic monitoring systems for at least 1 month. Interestingly, during the period of observation the overall compliance was greater than 80% in 33 patients and serious problems of non-adherence were found in only four patients. Yet a significant improvement of the efficacy of drug therapies was observed in 50% of patients, suggesting that non-compliance was more common without the use of electronic monitoring. A questionnaire was completed by patients, pharmacists and physicians to examine the impact of the monitoring system on the patient–physician, patient–pharmacist and pharmacist–physician relationships. The network significantly ameliorated the physician–pharmacist relationships, without affecting contact with the patient. These preliminary results indicate that the electronic monitoring of drug compliance, involving the physician as the prescriber and the pharmacist as the service provider, is probably very useful to improve the overall drug adherence. Larger, controlled clinical studies should now be performed to examine the economic and medical impacts of this network.

ON-LINE ELECTRONIC MONITORING OF HIGH-RISK PATIENTS

The precise cost of non-compliance is difficult to calculate because existing data are limited and approximated. Yet if one assumes that the compliance rate is as low as 50% for most chronic diseases such as hypertension, hyperlipidemia, epilepsy or heart failure, the potential for savings could be enormous[17,18]. The cost of non-compliance is particularly high when missing several drug doses can result in an emergency admission to the hospital, as is the case, for example, for epilepsy or congestive heart failure. For some of these high-risk patients, a closer day-to-day monitoring of drug compliance may be more appropriate to prevent additional hospital admissions.

The MEMS Dosing Partners Program (Aprex Corporation, Fremont, California, USA) has been developed for this purpose to help elderly people who have difficulty in remembering medication doses or patients taking medicines that could lead to serious medical problems if not taken regularly[4]. This program consists of a MEMS unit combined with a small, portable modem that transmits data every night from the patient's home to a central computer at the physician's office or in a pharmacy. When missed doses or inappropriate dose intervals are noted, direct contact with the patient can be established by trained compliance counsellors (the physician, a pharmacist or a nurse). No data have yet been published on the efficacy and acceptability of this approach. Since patients may object to intrusions of privacy we have recently studied the acceptability of this system in Switzerland in a small group of patients (seven) aged 35–74 (mean 58) years with uncomplicated chronic diseases[28]. Three patients were taking an oral antidiabetic agent (metformin, two or three daily doses), one patient a lipid-regulating agent (simvastatin, one daily dose) and three an antihypertensive agent (enalapril, nifedipine and felodipine, one daily dose). The study was conducted in two phases. For one month, each patient received his usual medicine in an electronic monitor to measure the baseline drug compliance. At the end of this period, a modem connected to the pharmacist's computer was installed on the patient's telephone line. During the next month, the patient was asked to put down his monitor on the modem every evening. At the end of the study, each patient completed a questionnaire to evaluate the acceptability of the modem. Technically, no particular problem was found. Less than 5% (13/265) of the modem calls failed and no data was lost. The patients' phone lines were engaged by the modem every night for 12–19 seconds, depending on the size of the message, representing only a marginal cost for telephone calls. Four of the seven patients were very good compliers throughout the study (>95% days with correct dosing). The other three had a low global baseline compliance with the MEMS but their compliance improved during the modem period, from a mean of 76% to 89%. These three patients stated in the questionnaire that the program helped them take their pills regularly.

The modem was well accepted by the patients. Its small size and the fact that the instrument is silent and never occupies the connection when the patient wanted to use the phone were considered as positive. The location of the modem at home was judged very important by all the patients although it was sometimes felt as a limitation. Ideally, it should be placed in a quiet, safe and accessible room, close to the other medicines. The modem was rarely perceived as an intruding tool as long as the reasons for installing it were correctly explained. Telephone interventions were rare but particularly delicate as tact was required; the pharmacist or the physician needed to listen carefully to the patient to try to understand the drug behavior problem and to propose a solution. The conclusion of this preliminary study is that on-line monitoring of home drug compliance is not only technically but also practically feasible and acceptable by the patients when correctly explained. This system could be used in some occasions as an interactive, instructive and educative instrument, especially for high-risk patients. We are now studying the efficacy and cost-effectiveness of this system in epileptic patients with a high incidence of crisis.

CONCLUSIONS

Non-compliance is a well documented clinical problem that is still far from being solved. Despite the various strategies commonly proposed to enhance drug adherence, little progress has been made in the last 10 years[29,30]. This relative failure to improve compliance has several causes, the most important of which is the quality of the detection procedures, which are generally inadequate and tedious and hence not applied. In addition, except for some simple recommendations regarding the dose regimens, personalized counseling for compliance (which is time-consuming) is rarely provided. The lack of objective data for discussion certainly contributes to the absence of dialogue. Finally, physicians and pharmacists have no feedback on the patient's behavior and few of these care providers have received specific training in compliance management.

A wider use of microelectronic monitoring systems in clinical practice may completely change our approach to compliance, providing new and precise information that no other monitoring system can produce. Computer-generated compliance reports are simple to prepare and rapidly available, enabling immediate feedback discussion with patients. Today, the electronic monitoring of compliance is the best and most reliable method of assessing compliance and should be used as the reference method. However, single-intervention strategies have rarely been effective, particularly during long-term treatment, and the use of electronic monitoring should therefore be combined with other interventions such as reminders, educational programs, information brochures or behavioral strategies (Table 6.3). Since compliance is a dynamic parameter, monitoring may be prescribed either continuously or periodically. In any case, monitoring should always be used in a mutually agreeable treatment plan developed within a patient–professional partnership. Effective healthcare provider networks should be created to achieve significant improvements in the management of compliance based on

TABLE 6.3 Potential causes of non-compliance and possible interventions for improving drug adherence

Potential causes of non-compliance	Possible interventions
Non-acceptability	
Refusal of diagnosis. Refusal of treatment (personal beliefs)	Better communication between the patient and the physician or other healthcare provider. Negotiation of the treatment plan
Non-comprehension	
Insufficient comprehension of the disease and the treatment. Insufficient understanding of the risk/benefit ratio	Improve communication between patient and healthcare provider
Problems with medication	
Side-effects, size of the pills, taste, number of doses a day	Modification and simplification of treatment regimen
Forgetfulness	
Forgetfulness due to age, stress, lack of motivation etc., bad integration of the drug into daily life	Association of the pill taking with a daily activity, family support, modification or simplification of the treatment, technical help—such as a daily dose reminder, an electronic monitoring system with an electronic window, a pager, permanent contact through a modem, telephone calls

electronic monitoring. We need no more studies showing that patient compliance is poor: rather, large, well designed prospective studies should be conducted to demonstrate cost-effectiveness and the clinical benefits of the new monitoring systems on the patient's outcome.

Acknowledgements

This work was supported by a grant from the Drug Information Association and by Pfizer AG, Switzerland.

REFERENCES

1. Urquhart J. Patient compliance with prescribed drug regimens: overview of the past 30 years of research. In: *Clinical Measurement in Drug Evaluation*. WS Nimmo, GT Tucker, eds. John Wiley & Sons, 1995; pp. 213–227
2. Sackett DL, Snow JC. The magnitude of adherence and nonadherence. In: Haynes RB, Taylor DW, Sackett DL, eds. *Compliance in Health Care*. Baltimore:John Hopkins University Press, 1979; pp. 11–22
3. Stewart RB, Cluff LE. A review of medication errors and compliance in ambulant patients. *Clin Pharmacol Ther* **13**:463–468, 1972

4. Stockwell Morris LS, Schulz RM. Patient compliance—An overview. *J Clin Pharm Ther* 17:283–295, 1992
5. Cramer J.A. Microelectronic systems for monitoring and enhancing patient compliance with medication regimens. *Drugs* 49(3):321–327, 1995
6. Urquhart J. The electronic medication event monitoring. Lessons for pharmacotherapy. *Clin Pharmacokinet* 32(5):345–356, 1997
7. Cramer JA, Mattson RH, Prevey ML, Scheyer RD, Ouellette VL. How often is medication taken as prescribed ? A novel assessment technique. *JAMA* 261(22): 3273–3277, 1989
8. Elliott WJ. Compliance strategies. *Curr Opin Nephrol Hypertens* 3:271–278, 1994
9. Kruse W, Rampmaier J, Ullrich G, Weber E. Patterns of drug compliance with medications to be taken once and twice daily assessed by continuous electronic monitoring in primary care. *Int J Clin Pharmacol Ther* 32 (9):452–457, 1994
10. Waterhouse DM, Calzone KA, Mele C, Brenner DE. Adherence to oral tamoxifen: a comparison of patient self-report, pill counts, and microelectronic monitoring. *J Clin Oncol* 11:1189–1197, 1993
11. Guerrero D, Rudd P, Bryant-Kosling C, Middleton BF. Antihypertensive medication-taking. Investigation of a simple regimen. *Am J Hypertens* 6:586–592, 1993
12. Kruse W, Eggert-Kruse W, Rampmaier J, Runnerbaum B, Weber E. Compliance and adverse drug reactions: a prospective study with ethinylestradiol using continuous compliance monitoring. *Clin Invest* 71:483 487, 1993
13. Matsuyama JR, Mason BJ, Jue SG. Pharmacists' intervention using an electronic medication event monitoring device's adherence data versus pill counts. *Ann Pharmacother* 27:851 855, 1993
14. Kruse W, Koch GP, Nikolaus T, Oster P, Schlierf G, Weber E. Measurement of drug compliance by continuous electronic monitoring: a pilot study in elderly patients discharged from hospital. *J Am Geriatr Soc* 40:1151–1155, 1992
15. Kruse W, Nikolaus T, Rampmaier J, Weber E, Schlierf G. Actual versus prescribed timing of lovastatin doses assessed by electronic compliance monitoring. *Eur J Clin Pharmacol* 45:211–215, 1993
16. Matsui D, Hermann C, Klein J, Berkovitch M, Olivieri N, Koren G. Critical comparison of novel and existing methods of compliance assessment during a clinical trial of an oral iron chelator. *J Clin Pharmacol* 34:944–949, 1994
17. Murphy J, Coster G. Issues in patient compliance. *Drugs* 54(6):797–800, 1997
18. Rogers PG, Bullman R. Prescription medicine compliance: a review of the baseline of knowledge—a report of the National Council on Patient Information and Education. *J Pharmacoepidemiol* 3(2):3–36, 1995
19. Sackett DL, Haynes RB, Guyatt GH, Tugwell P. Helping patients follow the treatments you prescribe. In: *Clinical Epidemiology. A Basic Science For Clinical Medicine.* Second Edition. DL Sackett, RB Haynes, GH Guyatt and PT Tugwell, eds. Boston: Little, Brown & Co., 1991; pp. 249–281
20. Fallab-Stubi CL, Zellweger JP, Sauty A, Uldry Ch, Iorillo D, Burnier M. Electronic monitoring of adherence to treatment in the preventive chemotherapy of tuberculosis. *Int J Tuberc Lung Dis* 2(7):1–6, 1998
21. American Pharmaceutical Association. *A new outpatient pharmacy services benefit: achieving value from pharmacists services.* Washington, DC: American Pharmaceutical Association, 1994
22. Bond WS, Hussar DA. Detection and strategies for improving medication compliance. *Am J Hosp Pharm* 48:1978–1988, 1991

23. Lip GYH, Beevers DG. Doctors, nurses, pharmacists and patients—the rational evaluation and choice in hypertension (REACH) survey of hypertension care delivery. *Blood Press* **6** (suppl 1):6–10, 1997
24. Kravitz RL, Hays RD, Sherboune CD, DiMatteo R, Rogers WH, Ordway L, Greenfield S. Recall of recommendations and adherence to advice among patients with chronic medical conditions. *Arch Intern Med* **153**:1869–1878, 1993
25. Sackett DL, Haynes RB, Gibson ES, Hackett BC, Taylor DW, Roberts RS, Johnson AL. Randomised clinical trials of strategies for improving medication compliance in primary hypertension. *Lancet* **i**:1205–1207, 1975
26. Steiner JF, Prochazka AV. The assessment of refill compliance using pharmacy records: methods, validity, and applications. *J Clin Epidemiol* **50**(1):105–116, 1997
27. Garnett WR, Davis LR, McKenney JM, Steiner K. Effect of telephone follow-up on medication compliance. *Am J Hosp Pharm* **38**:676–679, 1981
28. Schneider MP, Burnier M. On-line home monitoring of drug compliance: is it feasible? *Eur J Clin Pharmacol* **54**(6):489–490, 1998
29. Haynes RB, McKibbon KA, Kanani R. Systematic review of randomised trials of interventions to assist patients to follow prescription for medications. *Lancet* **348**:383–386, 1996
30. Heidel B, Wiffen PJ. Improving patient compliance with medication: a review of randomised controlled trials. *EHP* **2**(1):13–16, 1996

7

Non-compliance and Clinical Trials: Regulatory Perspectives

Carl Peck

Center for Drug Development Science, Georgetown University Medical Center, Washington, DC

INTRODUCTION

Adherence of subjects in a clinical trial to the assigned drug treatment regimen is as much a determinant of outcomes of the trial as it is of influencing patients' therapeutic responses in the practice of medicine. In the past regulatory authorities have, by and large, ignored treatment non-compliance in evaluation of clinical trials of new drugs but recently some regulatory guidance documents have acknowledged the problem of non-compliance. In this chapter, regulatory authorities' attitudes towards non-compliance are considered and their implications for drug labeling and drug development are explored.

REGULATORY ATTITUDES REGARDING PATIENT NON-COMPLIANCE

Traditionally, attitudes of Western regulatory authorities regarding patient non-compliance, as reflected in published guidelines and practice, have appeared to be passive, or even resistant, with only exceptional inclusion of non-compliance considerations in actual drug labeling. Unfortunately, due to the conformist nature of the strongly regulated research pharmaceutical industry, these attitudes are mimicked by practitioners of registration clinical trials. Nevertheless, regulatory attitudes appear to be changing in the direction of greater recognition of compliance as a factor to be considered in several aspects of drug development and regulatory review.

Until recently few, if any, regulatory guidelines for industry specifically addressed the issue of non-compliance in registration clinical trials. However, a few FDA guidelines and guidances now acknowledge the non-compliance

Drug Regimen Compliance: Issues in Clinical Trials and Patient Management.
Edited by J.-M. Métry and U.A. Meyer. © 1999 John Wiley & Sons Ltd.

problem in the following contexts: drug container closure systems (e.g. compliance barriers due to difficult to open pill bottle caps)[1], listing compliance assessment methods in clinical study reports[2], general considerations for methods to reduce or assess bias in clinical trials[3], and statistical principles for clinical trials[4].

Unfortunately, acknowledgment does not reflect adequate encouragement or guidance on use of modern methods of compliance testing. For example, the Center for Drug Development Science[5] found the ICH E9 draft document 'Guideline on Statistical Principles for Clinical Trials' generally deficient in its lack of consideration of medication non-compliance and, specifically, in its discouragement of compliance assessments via emphasis on employment of the intention-to-treat (ITT) policy. While individual clinical guidelines may acknowledge the phenomenon of imperfect adherence to assigned treatments or may even suggest (biased) compliance assessment methods such as pill counts, the regulatory view has generally been to consciously ignore treatment non-compliance along with other protocol violations by demanding employment of the ITT policy. This policy, applied to the analysis of completed clinical trials in an effort to preserve all randomized treatment assignments, essentially forces statistical hypothesis testing of all cases that were entered into the trial, regardless of treatment protocol errors committed during the trial (including missed or wrongly timed doses, unassigned doses and premature cessation of treatment). Moreover, no regulatory guidance on how to incorporate compliance assessments into the analysis of clinical trials has been forthcoming. In effect, the lack of encouragement by regulatory authorities, their receptivity to inadequate compliance assessment methods, and wholesale discounting of compliance data via the ITT policy, has been interpreted by the research pharmaceutical industry as active resistance to incorporation and utilization of compliance data in registration trials, documents and labeling.

Thus, it could be concluded that regulatory authorities have largely undervalued non-compliance. However, that is not entirely the case. A recent regulatory review policy reflected in a guidance to reviewers[6] drew attention to medication compliance as a criterion for establishing priority for reviews of registration documents. The 1996 US FDA review priority policy states that 'documented enhancement of patient compliance' is a sufficient criterion for establishing a 'P–Priority review'. This review priority level is limited to drug applications that 'have the potential for providing significant preventive or diagnostic therapeutic advance as compared to "standard" applications'[6].

A temporary exception to the lack of attention to non-compliance was the US drug label for cholestyramine[7], which listed as risk reduction factors the observed coronary heart disease risk reduction according to dosage levels actually ingested that were inferred from pill counts of subjects in the Lipid Research Clinics Coronary Primary Prevention Trial[8]: risk reduction in poor compliers was 11% whereas it was 40% in full compliers (ITT estimate was

19%). This information was first included in the cholestyramine label in January 1985 but was removed for unexplained reasons in the September 1995 revision.

Nevertheless, a model of informative and helpful labeling for women who miss one or more daily birth control pills can be found in the US class labeling for oral contraceptives[9]. Detailed patient labeling warns that 'the chance of becoming pregnant increases with each missed pill during the menstrual cycle.' Explicit instructions are given for actions to be taken when one or more pills are missed in order to avoid contraceptive failure.

CLINICAL IMPLICATIONS OF NON-COMPLIANCE IN REGISTRATION CLINICAL TRIALS

Non-compliance in clinical trials has implications for both drug efficacy and safety. When the principal objective of a registration clinical trial is simply to establish whether a new drug is effective or not, ignoring non-compliance and interpreting trial results according to the ITT policy may suffice, although the statistical power of such trials is impaired and dose–response patterns may be obscured. However, the amount or extent of effectiveness estimated in this fashion is diluted because subjects exhibiting partial or complete non-compliance are included in the analysis of trial results. Thus, the effectiveness is underestimated for full compliers with a prescribed drug regimen and the expected benefit for poor compliers is overestimated.

A more serious error ensues on the question of safety. As the data from partial or non-compliers contribute to the incidence of adverse reactions, safety may be underestimated by the inclusion of cases not fully exposed to the new drug. As in the case of efficacy, dose-related patterns of toxicity may be ambiguous. In addition, certain patterns of non-compliance such as drug holidays (multiple, consecutive missed doses), if they are not specifically identified may lead to special safety risks such as rebound or withdrawal toxicities. The implications of this biased, compliance-ignorant approach to safety assessment is that physicians prescribing a drug to full compliers may expect lower toxicity than is actually being risked, and the risks of missed doses may go undetected.

ARE DRUGS MISLABELED WHEN NON-COMPLIANCE IS IGNORED?

Currently approved drug labels provide data on safety and effectiveness according to clinical trial standards that have rarely included attention to non-compliance patterns. Although the effectiveness of such approved drugs is not in question, the precision of the labels in providing estimates of the effectiveness in a recipient of the recommended dosage may be poor, especially in a fully compliant patient. Greater than expected effectiveness is more tolerable, however, than unexpected side-effects or understated toxicity. Thus, while the traditional drug label may fulfill the legal requirement for regulatory confirmation of effectiveness and safety on a population scale, it serves the individual prescriber and recipient patient poorly by inadequately predicting individual outcome of therapy. Lasagna and Hutt[10] assert that any drug labeled for efficacy on the basis of compliance-ignorant ITT averages is mislabeled, technically, because the consequences of taking the recommended dosage are untruthfully described. Instead the label describes the average consequences of taking a lower dosage, which is the 'all-patient average' drug intake. This regulatory anomaly reflects a conflict between a full-disclosure labeling policy and statistical analytic policy.

REGULATORY ENCOURAGEMENT FOR DEVELOPMENT OF NON-COMPLIANCE FORGIVING DRUGS

One solution to the myriad problems associated with non-compliance in clinical trials is deliberate investigation of the consequences, if any, on safety and effectiveness of a drug deliberately or naturally subjected to typical non-compliance patterns. Clinical trials were first performed in the field of contraceptive therapeutics[11–15] in the late 1970s and early 1980s but some years elapsed before reports of clinical trials employing deliberate medication omissions appeared in another field (e.g. antihypertensive therapy[16–19]). Notably, no reports of clinical trials incorporating this procedure in the pre-market phase have been published. However, a recent trade press publication described a presentation before a FDA Advisory Committee of a pre-market clinical trial that employed 'simulated non-compliance' of the antihypertensive drug tasosartan[20]. Tasosartan, an angiotensin-II inhibitor which gives rise to two human metabolites with half-lives exceeding 2 days, retained adequate antihypertensive effects during chronic therapy despite 2 days of missed doses.

Conditions that favor persistent safety and effectiveness of drugs in the face of missed doses include a duration of action that far exceeds the plasma half-life or dosing interval (e.g. omeprazole: half-life 30 minutes, dosed once a day, duration of action more than 3 days) or long half-lives of parent compound or active metabolite(s) relative to the dosing interval such as fluoxetine (parent drug plasma half-life 7 days, half-life of active metabolite 18 days, dosage once a day) and tasosartan (see above). Such drugs may be considered non-compliance 'forgiving' in that occasionally missed doses do not result in lost effectiveness or safety problems. Regulatory agencies would in effect encourage development of such drugs if they insisted upon assessments of naturally occurring non-compliance or investigation of consequences of deliberate dosage cessation patterns.

REFERENCES

1. Guidance for Industry. *Submission of Documentation in Drug Applications for Container Closure Systems Used for Packaging of Human Drugs and Biologics.* US DHHS, FDA, CDER, CBER, June 1997, p. 10.
2. *Guideline for Industry. Structure and Content of Clinical Study Reports.* US FDA, International Conference on Harmonization of Technical Requirements for Registration of Pharmaceuticals for Human Use (ICH), E3, July 1996, pp. 16, 17, 22, 37.
3. *ICH Harmonized Tripartite Guideline. General Considerations for Clinical Trials.* US FDA, International Conference on Harmonization of Technical Requirements for Registration of Pharmaceuticals for Human Use (ICH), E6. Recommended for Adoption at Step 4 of the ICH Process on 17 July 1997, p. 11.
4. *Draft Consensus Guideline. Statistical Principles for Clinical Trials.* US FDA International Conference on Harmonization of Technical Requirements for Registration of Pharmaceuticals for Human Use (ICH), E6. Released for Consultation at Step 2 of the ICH Process on 16 January 1997, pp. 8, 23.
5. Peck CC. *Center for Drug Development Science Commentary on ICH E9 Draft Guideline on Statistical Principles for Clinical Trials,* July 3 1997. CDDS, Georgetown University, Washington, DC.
6. Review Management, Priority Review Policy. *Manual of Policies and Procedures (MAPP 6020.3).* US DHHS, FDA, CDER, CBER, April 4 1996, p. 2.
7. *Physicians Desk Reference,* 44th Edition. Medical Economics Co. Inc., Oradell, NJ, 1990, p. 727.
8. Anon. The Lipid Research Clinics Coronary Primary Prevention Trial results: (I) Reduction in incidence of coronary heart disease, (II) The relationship of reduction in incidence of coronary heart disease to cholesterol lowering. *JAMA* 1984; **251**:351–374.
9. *Physicians Desk Reference,* 51st Edition. Medical Economics Co. Inc., Oradell, NJ, 1997, pp. 2855–2857.
10. Lasagna L, Hutt BB. Health Care, Research, and Regulatory Impact of Non-compliance. In: *Patient Compliance in Medical Practice and Clinical Trials,* J. Cramer and B. Spilker, eds. Raven Press, NY, 1991, pp. 401–402.
11. Morris SE, Groom GV, Cameron ED, Buckingham MS, Everitt JM, Elstein M. Studies on low dose oral contraceptives: plasma hormone changes in relation to deliberate pill ('MICROGYNON-30') omission. *Contraception* 1979; **20**: 61–69.
12. Chowdry V, Joshi UM, Gopalkrishna K, Betrabet S, Mehta S, Saxena BN. 'Escape' ovulation in women due to the missing of low dose combination oral contraceptive pills. *Contraception* 1980; **22**: 241–247.
13. Wang E, Shi S, Cekan SZ, Landgren B-M, Diczfalusy E. Hormonal consequences of 'missing the pill'. *Contraception* 1982; **26**: 545–566.
14. Landgren B-M, Diczfalusy E. Hormonal consequences of missing the pill during the first two days of three consecutive artificial cycles. *Contraception* 1984; **29**: 437–446.
15. Smith SK, Kirkman RJE, Arce BB, McNeilly AS, Loudon NB, Baird DT. The effect of deliberate omission of TRINORDIOL or MICROGYNON on the hypothalamo-pituitary-ovarian axis. *Contraception* 1986; **34**: 513–522.
16. Johnson BF, Whelton A. A study design for comparing the effects of missing daily doses of antihypertensive drugs. *Am J Ther* 1994; **1**: 260–267.
17. Vaur L, Dutrey-Dupagne C, Boussac J. *et al.* Differential effects of a missed dose of trandolapril and enalapril on blood pressure control in hypertensive patients. *J Cardiovasc Pharmacol* 1995; **26**: 127–131.

18. Leenen FHH, Fourney A, Notman G, Tanner J. Persistence of anti-hypertensive effect after 'missed doses' of calcium antagonist with long (amlodipine) vs short (diltiazem) elimination half-life. *Br J Clin Pharmacol* 1996; **41**: 83–88.

19. Hernandez-Hernandez R, Armas de Hernandez MJ, Armas-Padilla MC, Carvajal AR, Guerrero-Pajuelo J. The effects of missing a dose of enalapril versus amlodipine on ambulatory blood pressure. *Blood Pressure Monitoring* 1996; 1: 1121–1126.

20. F-D-C Reports (*The Pink Sheet*). February 2 1998, p. 4.

8

Regulatory Issues

Jean-Marc Husson

*International Federation of the Associations of Pharmaceutical Physicians (IFAPP),
32 Avenue Duquesne, Paris, France*

INTRODUCTION

The pharmaceutical industry is probably the most regulated industry in the world; whatever the country, there is today the fear of a new disaster such as the one which involved thalidomide during the early 1960s.

However, in this context of possible over-regulation, the question of patient compliance with medicinal drugs is of particular importance because the place offered to it in most regulatory texts is apparently so small, or so vague, that patient compliance with drug could be today considered as an 'orphan regulatory request'. Paradoxically, when a new medicinal product is pre-scribed after its approval by regulatory authorities very little is known about its real safety and effectiveness. For most non-parenteral products, nobody knows whether the absence of response of a specific subject to a specific dose for a specific indication is due to the fact that the patient is a non-responder or a non-complier.

The purpose of this chapter is to review where, when and how patient compliance could impact regulatory request during clinical development, evaluation/approval and post-marketing use of new medicines. This question is essential for all those involved in and interested by medicinal products: study subjects, patients, regulatory authorities, the pharmaceutical industry, and health professionals.

The precise measurement of patient compliance is a very serious matter and an important tool for at least three reasons:

1. Whatever the quality assurance system involved in the clinical develop-ment of a new drug, the poor measurement of patient compliance could adversely affect protection of study subject, the intrinsic quality of the clinical data and the integrity of that data (detection of possible fraud and misconduct).

Drug Regimen Compliance: Issues in Clinical Trials and Patient Management.
Edited by J.-M. Métry and U.A. Meyer. © 1999 John Wiley & Sons Ltd.

2. The poor control of patient compliance during clinical development could have a negative impact on the evaluation and subsequent labeling of the new medicinal product by regulatory authorities. In other words, in the final assessment of dosage and dose regimen.
3. Any mislabeling of a drug at the time of its approval could have a negative impact during marketing, on clinical safety (by overdosing) or therapeutic response (by underdosing). Correct measurement of patient compliance with drug, allowing a better knowledge of the clinical safety and effectiveness of the medicinal product, can lead to a more rational use of drugs.

The patient cannot be considered as 'guilty' of non-compliance. Most patients who are prescribed and delivered a medicinal product by health professionals are, without proper training and direction on their use, partial compliers. This doesn't mean that the regulatory authorities and pharmaceutical industry must not assume responsibility for non-compliance, but they must take into account the importance of study subject compliance during clinical development of a drug and ensure that patients are educated in their use.

PATIENT COMPLIANCE WITH DRUG AND UPDATE ON INTERNATIONAL REGULATORY TEXTS

Preliminary Remarks

Patient compliance is, for most people, only a part of regulatory compliance, which is a must and has a special meaning in many countries. Regulatory compliance means the existence of a quality assurance system and involves many people insuring that the professionals concerned with development, registration, manufacturing etc. of medicines are following (and not infringing) the regulatory demand, especially in the fields of good practice (good laboratory practice (GLP), good manufacturing practice (GMP) and good clinical practice (GCP)). The counterpart to the industry/CRO quality assurance system on the side of the regulatory authorities is the need for inspection.
Patient compliance is thus not really an autonomous entity and is not given the importance it should have. Whether they are a complier or a non-complier with prescribed drugs, a study subject is not legally responsible for his or her behavior during research on medical products.

ICH Guidelines and Patient Compliance

The International Conference on Harmonisation (ICH) is a process involving the regulatory authorities and pharmaceutical industry in the European Union, Japan and the USA, referring to common technical requirements for (development and) registration of pharmaceuticals for human use in these three regions. The ICH concerns the content and format of the quality, safety and efficacy parts of the registration dossier of new medicinal products.

When trying to find out the importance of patient compliance for the ICH partners, it is of interest to review the content of the tripartite efficacy guidelines which have been published as part of regulatory texts, and to see whether or not the term 'compliance with drug' is really taken into consideration. Twelve different guidelines have been drafted and most have reached the ICH Step 4, leading to official publication of the texts and their implementation in the three regions (Table 8.1). These guidelines constitute the basis for a global clinical development plan and acceptance of foreign clinical data by the regulatory authorities of the ICH regions.

General Guidelines

Only some of the ICH Efficacy guidelines have a possible link with the question of patient compliance with drug. All of them concern the clinical development process and the technical content of the clinical documentation for registration—with the exception of E3, which covers the 'structure and

TABLE 8.1 ICH Efficacy guidelines and patient compliance with medicinal products

Regulatory domains	Technical requirements	ICH efficacy guidelines	Reference to patient compliance with drug
Generalities	General considerations for clinical trials	E8[1]	None?
Reliability of data protection of subjects	GCP	E6[2]	Yes?
Methodology and technical requirements	Dose response	E4[3]	None
	Long-term exposure	E1[4]	None
	Safety reports	E2, A,B,C[5–7]	None
	Geriatrics	E7[8]	None
	Choice of control groups	E10[9]	None
	Statistical considerations	E9[10]	Yes?
Structure and content	Clinical study report	E3[11]	Yes
Acceptability of foreign data	Ethnic factors	E5[12]	Yes

content of the clinical study report'. However, there is still a long way to go, before changing the attitude of both regulatory authorities and industry in term of real measurement and statistical consideration of patient compliance with drug.

The framework or umbrella of all ICH Efficacy Guidelines, Guideline E8, covers the general considerations for clinical trials. By itself, it does not contain a precise reference to compliance with drug, and the ICH Efficacy glossary (a future appendix to E8) will contain only the term 'regulatory compliance' (Figure 8.1).

The guideline on GCP, E6, contains many references to compliance (in relation to trials) or to non-compliance issues, either within the guideline itself or within the glossary, but the term 'compliance with drug' (or medicinal product) is never mentioned. For example, in the part referring to the investigator it is said (paragraph 4.6.6): 'The investigator, or a person designated by the investigator/institution, should explain the correct use of the Investigational product(s) to each subject and should check, at intervals appropriate for the trial, that each subject is following the instructions properly'.

This is only vague advice on patient compliance with drug to regulatory compliers. The acronym GCP could cover the best or the worst of clinical practice depending on the quality assurance system which supports it, but this necessary regulatory requirement covers insufficiently, if at all, the question of patient compliance. GCP could also mean 'good compliance practice' and for this simple reason the health professionals who stress the importance of both quality and scientific aspects of patient compliance are correct in their approach.

Guideline E5, 'Ethnic factors in the acceptability of foreign clinical data', is one of the most innovative ICH guidelines. 'Ethnic factors' are defined in this document as those factors relating to the genetic and physiologic (intrinsic), and cultural and environmental (extrinsic) characteristics of a population. One reference on 'drug compliance' is made in Table 8.2 (appendix A to the E5 text) among extrinsic ethnic factors to be considered when evaluating the impact of these factors upon a drug's effect on a target population (i.e. its efficacy and safety at a particular dosage and dose regimen).

Target Population Guidelines

Among the populations at risk of poor compliance, elderly patients are easily disposed to poor compliance and the consequences linked to either under- or overdosing. Compliance of elderly patients is not even mentioned in Guideline E7 'Special populations: Geriatrics'. A new guideline (E11) is being drafted to cover children, but so far no other ICH guideline covers other populations at risk.

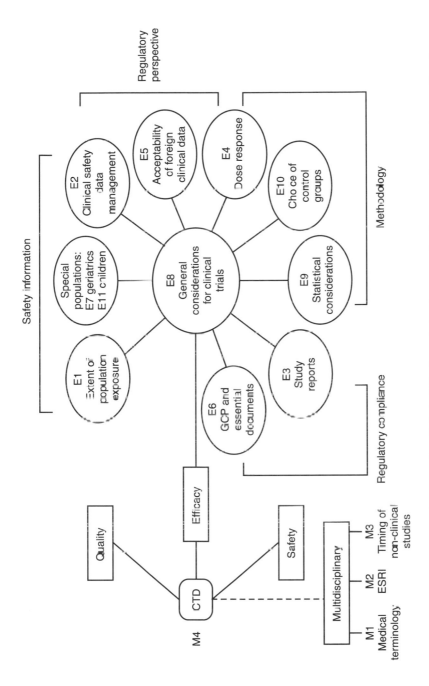

FIGURE 8.1 General considerations for clinical trials. Correlation between development phases and type of study

TABLE 8.2 Classification of intrinsic and extrinsic ethnic factors

	Intrinsic	Extrinsic
Genetic	Physiological and pathological conditions	Environmental
Gender	Age (children–elderly) Liver, kidney, cardiovascular functions	Climate: sunlight, pollution Culture: socioeconomic factors, education/training, language
Height	Diseases	Ethics: Medical practice, disease definition/diagnosis, therapeutic approach, drug compliance
Body weight	Smoking, alcohol consumption	Regulatory practice/GCP
ADME receptor sensitivity	Food habits	Methodology/endpoints
Race	Stress	
Genetic polymorphism of drug metabolism		
Genetic diseases		

Clinical Safety Guidelines

The text E1, on 'The extent of population exposure to assess clinical safety for long-term use of drugs prescribed in non-life-threatening conditions' does not mention patient compliance. Is it possible to measure the real safety profile of a drug without seriously taking into consideration and measuring patient compliance with medicinal products?

The series of guidelines on 'Clinical Safety Data Management' are among the good achievements of ICH, because they not only harmonize the expedited reporting of adverse events (ADEs: E2A) or adverse drug reactions (ADRs) and periodic safety updates (E2C) but also rationalize the approach to reporting (E2B). The question of compliance is implicit in the difference between adverse reaction and ADE, but there is no real request to measure and control compliance.

Methodological Guidelines

Guideline E4 refers to dose response studies for the development of new medicinal products. This important, but rather academic, text entirely ignores the question of compliance. These clinical exploratory studies are, however, key in defining the dosage and regimen for new medicinal products, whatever the methodology used.

The guideline on statistical principles for clinical trials, E9, should be one of the key texts on the question of patient compliance but, in fact, the intent to treat (ITT) dogma (called in this guideline 'Analysis of All Randomised Patients') is still the intangible statistical approach for regulatory authorities for planning, analysing and interpreting clinical trials on medicinal products. The 'Per Protocol' analysis is, however, considered as a complementary possibility and the guideline mentions indirectly the question of patient compliance with drug.

Guideline E10, 'Choice of Control Groups' very ambitiously tries to rationalize the selection of reference products (placebo and active substances) for clinical exploratory (phases II A and B) and confirmatory studies (phase III). The question of patient compliance is not considered in this important text.

The introduction of elements on compliance with drug will have to be reconsidered when these methodological guidelines are updated (ICH maintenance phase).

The Clinical Dossier

Guideline E3 refers to the structure and content of the clinical study report and is the only ICH document to have specific paragraphs and an appendix on compliance. Paragraph 9.4.8 on treatment compliance states: 'The measures taken to ensure and document Treatment Compliance should be described; e.g. drug accountability, diary cards, blood, urine and other body fluids drug level measurements or medication event monitoring.'

Measurements of treatment compliance are dealt with in paragraph 11.3: 'Any measurement of compliance of individual patients with the treatment regimen under study and drug concentrations in body fluid, should be summarised and analysed by treatment group and time interval and tabulated in Appendix 16.2.5.'

Appendix 16.2.5 stipulates that 'Patient data listing on compliance and/or drug concentration data should be available'.

The clinical study report (CSR) will, in the near future, be integrated in one ICH 'Common Technical Document' (CTD), officially accepted by the ICH Steering Committee as topic M4, which will simplify the preparation and the submission of the documentation for marketing authorization application/ new drug application (MAA/NDA) in the three ICH regions. The clinical part of the CTD dossier will cover written and tabulated summaries, essential parts of the registration dossier. Patient compliance will have to be considered as much as in the CSR. For these reasons, what is taken into account in the CSR (and subsequently the CTD) will be reconsidered in future methodological guidelines (E4, E9, E10).

TO COMPLY OR NOT TO COMPLY: WHERE ARE THE PROBLEMS?

When considering patient compliance during drug development, several questions must be successively answered:

1. Is the study subject/patient a complier or a non-complier?
2. In case of a negative therapeutic outcome, is the subject a non-complier or a non-responder?
3. Is the patient at risk:
   (a) elderly or young?
   (b) covered or not by a health care system?
   (c) suffering from a life-threatening or disabling disease?
4. Reasons for prescription and delivery of the medicinal product:
   (a) what are its therapeutic indications: high-risk population (organ transplant, epilepsy, AIDS, tuberculosis, type II diabetes, hypertension) or others?
   (b) in which pharmaceutical form (e.g. oral, spray) is it supplied?
   (c) is it designed for prophylactic or curative treatment?
   (d) is treatment short or long term?

There is no simple rule, no single answer, to these questions—but compliance must be handled carefully, whatever the population at risk. There are in fact two situations, which are totally different:

1. Compliance issues during the clinical development of a new medicinal product, before the application of the registration dossier, which have consequences on the evaluation process and approval by regulatory authorities.
2. Compliance problems following MAA/NDA labeling and their consequences on clinical safety and effectiveness, concerning the target population(s), according to the drug labeling/summary of medicinal product characteristics (officially SPC).

TOOLS FOR MONITORING PATIENT COMPLIANCE: A REGULATORY OR TECHNICAL PROBLEM?

Many techniques have been used to monitor compliance and to help patients to comply with directions for drug use (Table 8.3).

The positive and negative aspects of these techniques are described elsewhere in this book. The microelectronic monitoring systems are by far the most reliable of all these tools: they do not prove ingestion/intake of orally prescribed drugs, but have the unique advantages of counting the number of pills taken, the interval between doses and detection of holiday patterns, with their consequences.

TABLE 8.3   Techniques of monitoring patient compliance with drug

Patient self-observation (e.g. diary card)
Periodic pill count (the dogma for most authorities in the world)
Chemical markers in body fluids
Radioactive tracers
Review of pharmacy records
Electronic time monitoring systems (e.g. electronic drug event monitoring)

The time event monitoring system is the only technique to ensure the three 'Basic Principles' of GCP:

1. The protection of patients (by controlling patient over- or undercompliance).
2. The quality of clinical data (by facilitating patient monitoring and management of both clinical safety and efficacy data).
3. The integrity and reliability of clinical data (by preventing and detecting fraud and misconduct in clinical research by health professionals.

However, mastering such an electronic system is a very demanding and time consuming exercise.

The medication event monitoring system cannot guarantee by itself that the drug removed from its container has been swallowed/ingested, but other techniques such as control of compliance by chemical markers of body fluids, could also be artificially modified by patients.

In summary, there is no absolute tool to monitor patient compliance with drug, especially in long-term treatment, but electronic event monitoring systems are the most reliable.

Physician Prescription of Drugs and Patient Compliance with Directions for Use

As described by Lasagna and Hutt[13], non-compliance can take four different forms:

1. Taking more medicine than has been prescribed (overcompliance leading to overdosing).
2. Taking less medicine than prescribed, or none (undercompliance leading to underdosing).
3. Modifying the times and intervals of medicine intakes, possibly leading to holiday patterns with their possible rebound and recurrent first-dose effects.
4. Taking the medicine under contraindicated conditions (time/type of meals), in conjunction with other (unauthorized) medicines, possibly

entailing clinically significant drug/drug interactions. This questionable patient practice could induce a clinical safety problem (e.g. serious adverse drug reaction) or a negative therapeutic outcome (which is different from a non-response).

The absence of consideration for patient compliance can lead to a mislabeling of the involved drug, possibly risking a public health problem. After marketing authorization the case is more individual (the non-complier patient is the individual victim), even if the public health authorities are still concerned by the matter of any pharmacovigilance problems.

Patient non-compliance depends on many factors, such as

- Cultural or social level (education, profession, income)
- Psychological profile
- Environmental factors (e.g. family, friends, etc)

but can also be a consequence of

- Type of disease
- Patient confidence in his/her physician (contact, follow-up, diagnosis, treatment)
- Therapeutic approach (number of drugs, complexity and convenience of treatments)
- Absence of education on use of the drug
- Absence of real effectiveness of treatment (improvement, quality of life)
- Appearance of ADEs.

No real figures are available on patient compliance during clinical development or after marketing approval, but it is estimated today[14] that 65–70% of patients are good compliers, 25–30% are poor compliers and only 5% are total non-compliers.

Regulatory Demand and Education of Patients/Healthy Subjects

Many techniques have been developed to improve compliance. These include

- Patient education as early as possible (in the family; at school)
- Written directions for use
- Greater involvement of pharmacists, nurses, and investigators
- Electronic monitoring systems
- Home programmes (e.g. Telecom, Internet).

In the last two cases, technical approaches partially fill in the gap with regulatory demand.

REGULATORY ISSUES

Patient Compliance During Clinical Development of a New Medicine (or a New Therapeutic Indication/Pharmaceutical Forum)

Facts

For regulatory authorities and sponsors, the first time patient compliance is taken into consideration during the life of a new drug is when the clinical development program starts. The development classically follows a stepwise approach (Figure 8.2), each development step depending entirely on the clinical safety and efficacy results of the previous one. It has been assumed (without precise figures) that patient compliance distribution during clinical development corresponds to that in daily clinical practice.

The absence of real monitoring of compliance during drug development could have serious consequences for the outcomes of all types of clinical studies, but are of crucial importance for key clinical trials (such as pharmacokinetic/pharmacodynamic (PK/PD) studies, dose response exploratory studies, pivotal confirmatory studies). It is difficult to define the dosage and regimen of a new medicine without monitoring precisely patient compliance.

Compliance with drug *must* be considered in the following stages:

- Planning of a clinical study (study design, statistical hypothesis, protocol, flow chart etc.).
- Selection of patients. The inclusion of study subjects could be predefined in the protocol according to the level of compliance—this point must be included in the protocol.
- Monitoring. The quality control process is generally not sufficient, and should be combined with an electronic monitoring system.
- Analysing data. New statistical tools, as mentioned in another chapter, will emerge to aid planning and analysis of the impact of non-compliance on safety and efficacy. The purpose of this new statistical approach is not to abolish ITT analysis but to prompt authorities to take into consideration and analyse the impact of compliance through a per protocol analysis.
- Reporting. The clinical study report, according to ICH E3, is the only regulatory text to take into account the importance of compliance, but at the moment does so more as wishful thinking than as a must for the statistical analysis of the study.
- Auditing. Checking and ensuring the protection of study subjects, the quality and the integrity of the data is really possible only with adequate monitoring of compliance. Compliance is the cornerstone of GCP procedures even if today the word 'compliance' defines, broadly speaking, regulatory compliance, compliance with the protocol or, more specifically, patient compliance with drug.

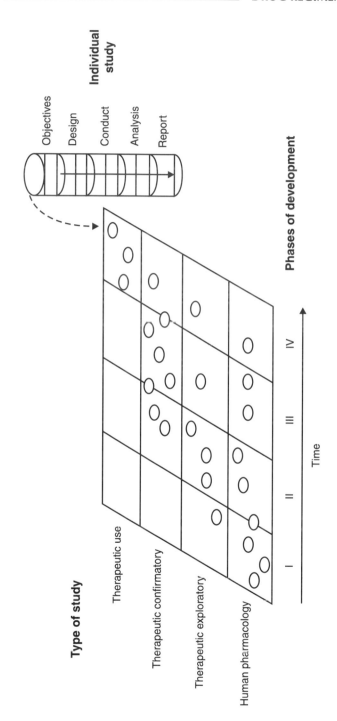

FIGURE 8.2 Achievements after ICH first phase (after ICH Guideline E8[*])

Absence of consideration of patient compliance is difficult to understand and must be further discussed.

Attitudes of Regulatory Bodies and Industry to Patient Non-compliance

The attitude of various bodies to patient non-compliance has been classified by Peck[15] as

1. Passive
2. Passive resistant
3. Exceptional

See Table 8.4. Regulatory authorities and industry are most often passive followers. They accept unreliable methods of measuring compliance (such as investigator checking, patient diary, pill count). They are reluctant to introduce non-requested methods and subsequently ignore the importance of compliance data.

Passive resistance is in most cases the 'politically correct' attitude: the ITT analysis is a dogma in planning, analysing, interpreting, and reporting clinical trials on drugs—even if ICH Guideline E9 half-opens the door to patient compliance interest within the context of the per protocol analysis. But ITT ignores drop-outs, missed doses/drug 'holidays' and their consequences (rebound and first-dose effect). The per protocol analysis is regarded by most statisticians as a bias. In summary there is no real wish, no 'leadership' (as said by Peck), to introduce compliance data in the statistical planning and analysis of clinical trials.

An exception concerns oral contraceptives, for which the authorities have decided to incorporate special directions in the labeling/product information. These outline the steps that the patient should take when the usual time for taking the daily contraceptive pill has passed without the pill having been taken, and only later has the patient realized either that she is late in taking the pill, or that she has omitted taking the pill for one or more days. This information is summarized by Guillebaud, along with a brief review of the scientific evidence that supports the recommendations. The information has come from studies in which placebo pills were substituted for active pills, to ascertain how soon the risk of ovulation, and thus of unwanted conception, begins to rise after the last-taken pill. As Guillebaud shows, the resulting data translate into a set of simple directions for the patient in order to: (a) minimize the risk of unwanted conception, and (b) make a safe and effective transition back to one-pill-a-day dosing. This new approach to labeling information is an important advance, especially in view of the fact that the oral contraceptives are collectively the most extensively used pharmaceutical products in history. This new labeling information for oral contraceptives is a

TABLE 8.4 Patient compliance with drugs and clinical trials: consequences on safety and efficacy regulatory issues

---

A: Regulatory (and industry) attitude to patient non-compliance

Passive:
1. Receptivity of unreliable methods (investigator, patient diary, pill count)
2. Reluctance to introduce non-requested methods
3. Compliance data largely discounted

Passive resistant:
1. ITT policy is a dogma in planning, analysing, interpreting clinical trials on drugs
2. ITT ignores drop-outs, missed doses (e.g. drug holiday pattern), per protocol analysis regarded as a bias
3. Lack of guidance on incorporation of compliance data in planning and analysis of clinical trials
4. No leadership, despite advances in statistics

One exception about labeling: the cholestyramine case

B: Statistical and regulatory implications of ITT policy:

1. Decreased power and increased sample size requirements
2. Failed trials (e.g. dose response)
3. Inaccurate estimates of safety/toxicity and effectiveness
4. Subsequent inaccurate labeling

C: Clinical implications of non-compliance (measurement) in clinical trials, in mislabeling:

Safety:
1. Risk underestimated by ITT strategy
2. Diluted estimation of toxicity incidence or severity
3. Real dose-related toxicity not described on drug label
4. Rebound (first-dose) effect toxicity due to holiday pattern

Efficacy:
1. Dose responsiveness obscured
2. Effectiveness not clearly estimated by ITT analysis, leading to inaccurate labeling on (hyper)efficacy, e.g. dose related, rebound, first-dose effect

---

After Peck[8]

model that all chronic-use pharmaceuticals should emulate, particularly since, as we now know, there is a prevalence of imperfect compliance in virtually every disease condition so far studied.

Regulatory Evaluation and Approval of a New Medicine

When the regulatory authorities assess a NDA/MAA dossier they are confronted with the absence of real measurements or knowledge of patient compliance. This can have consequences on the assessment/determination of safety, effectiveness and labeling of a new medicinal product.

Drug Effectiveness

The ITT analysis provides an *average* of effectiveness, but doesn't consider patient compliance and artificially increases type II errors. Consequently it decreases the power of the statistical hypothesis and increases sample size requirements. ITT overestimates the medicinal optimal dose, because it assumes that all patients are good compliers and accurately dosed. Even if individual titration rate has been used ITT does not show the *rate* of effectiveness, which stratifies and adjusts the patient compliance. The main consequence of ITT analysis, according to Peck, is to obscure dose response curves, leading to too many failed trials. This type of analysis also does not clearly estimate effectiveness, allowing inaccurate labeling on efficacy (rebound and first-dose effect).

Drug Safety

ITT underestimates the risk of toxicity, dilutes the incidence of severe adverse reactions, bypasses the real dose-related toxicity of the drug, misinterprets rebound or first-dose effects due to holiday pattern and misestimates the clinical safety profile of the new medicine. Every year drugs are withdrawn from the market for safety reasons due to:

1. The small size of the clinical database requested for approval, which does not offer the possibility to discover serious and rare adverse drug reactions.
2. The absence of real consideration of compliance during clinical development, which underestimates the potential toxic profile of the new medicine.

Drug Labeling

Mislabeling could be a consequence of ITT analysis unless precise analysis of patient compliance, planned in the protocol, is performed concurrently. Inaccurate estimates of effectiveness (due to an inadequate dose response curve), underestimation of toxicity incidence or severity, the absence of consideration of drug holidays (leading possibly to rebound and first-dose effects) are common sequelae of mislabeling. The assumption that the rate of non-compliance is the same after regulatory approval of a drug is not verified and doesn't have the same consequences on public health because this is rather the problem of an individual.

CONCLUSIONS

Patient compliance with medicinal products is today an 'orphan regulatory condition', because it is not seriously taken into consideration by regulatory authorities, the pharmaceutical industry and health professionals. There is still a long way to go to obtain the official recognition of the public health importance of patient compliance with drug.

Methods for measuring, controlling, and analysing compliance exist, but health professionals (especially statisticians from both authorities and industry/ CROs) deny its real importance, considering the problem in a very passive way. One day, GCP will also mean 'good compliance practice'. Poor compliance before MAA/NDA, could lead to mislabeling of a newly approved drug.

Following approval, poor patient compliance could induce, without proper patient education, serious individual problems such as severe adverse reactions or absence of a positive therapeutic outcome. Patient compliance is a permanent public health concern for health authorities. The challenge is to successfully transform an 'orphan' condition to daily practice.

REFERENCES

1. E8: Note for Guidance on General Conditions for Clinical Trials—CPMP/ ICH/291/9, Step 4.
2. E6: Explanatory note and comments to the ICH Harmonized Tripartite Guideline E6 – Note for Guidance on Good Clinical Practice – CPMP/ICH/768/97.
3. E4: Note for Guidance on Dose Response Information to support Drug Registration (CPMP adopted May 94) – CPMP/ICH/378/95).
4. E1: Note for Guidance on Population Exposure: the extent of Population Exposure to assess Clinical Safety (CPMP adopted November 94) – CPMP/ ICH/375/95.
5. E2A: Note for Guidance on Good Clinical Safety Data Management: Definitions and Standards for Expedited Reporting (CPMP adopted November 94) – CPMP/ ICH/377/95.
6. E2B: Note for Guidance on Clinical Safety Data Management: Data Elements for Transmission of Individual Case Safety Reports—CPMP/ICH/287/95.
7. E2C: Note for Guidance on Clinical Safety Data Management: Periodic Safety Update Reports for Marketed Drugs (CPMP adopted December 1995)—CPMP/ ICH/298/95.
8. E7: Note for Guidance on Studies in support of Special Populations: Geriatrics (CPMP adopted Sept. 93) – CPMP/ICH/379/95.
9. E10: The Choice of Control Groups—ICH Guideline, Step 2.
10. E9: Note for Guidance on Statistical Principles for Clinical Trials—CPMP/ ICH/363/96, Step 4.
11. E3: Note for Guidance on Structure and Content of Clinical Study Reports (CPMP adopted December 1995)—CPMP/ICH/136/95.
12. E5: Note for Guidance on Ethnic Factors in the Acceptability of Foreign Clinical Data—CPMP/ICH/289/95, Step 4 18.
13. Lasagna L, Hutt P. Health care, research, and regulatory impact of non-compliance. In JA Cramer, B Spilker (eds) _Compliance in Medical Practice and Clinical Trials._ New York: Raven Press, 1991, pp 393–403.
14. Urquhart J. The electronic medication event monitor – lessons for pharmacotherapy. _Clin Pharmacokinet_ **32**: 345–356, 1997.
15. Peck C. Non-compliance and clinical trials. Regulatory perspectives. In J-M Métry, UA Meyer (eds) _Drug Regimen Compliance: Issues in Clinical Trials and Patient Management._ Chichester: John Wiley & Sons Ltd., 1999, pp 97–102.

9

Pharmacoeconomic Impact of Variable Compliance

John Urquhart

Department of Epidemiology, Maastricht University, The Netherlands

INTRODUCTION

The advent of electronic monitoring has created a renaissance in research on patient non-compliance with prescribed drug regimens and with it has come new insight into the extent to which variable drug intake acts as a source of variance in drug response. The key advance that has brought about this renaissance is the ability to compile dosing histories of ambulatory patients by electronic monitoring (EM), based on the incorporation of time-stamping microcircuitry into drug packages, so as to provide a time-stamped record whenever the package is manipulated to remove a dose. The various forms that EM can take, and the assumptions upon which it is based and upon which package manipulation is interpreted as drug ingestion, are discussed by Urquhart[1] and in other chapters in this book.

EM is an important methodologic advance in several respects. First, it provides reliable data on the incidence and magnitude of deviations from prescribed drug regimens in ambulatory care. Second, it quantifies intervals between doses, enabling pharmacokinetic interpretation of actual versus prescribed dosing. Third, it provides information on *when* critical dosing errors occur, which is crucial for interpreting pharmacodynamic and clinical consequences of long lapses in dosing ('drug holidays') or other unusual patterns of dosing. Data from EM provide an objective answer to the question that is, or logically should be, prompted by inadequate response to ambulatory pharmacotherapy: pharmacological non-responder, poor bioavailability, or regimen non-complier?

The importance of this last point cannot be overstated. When a powerful drug is rationally prescribed, its subsequent action confirms the assumptions underlying the medical decision to prescribe it. These assumptions are challenged by partial or complete failure of the anticipated effect. A logical

Drug Regimen Compliance: Issues in Clinical Trials and Patient Management.
Edited by J.-M. Métry and U.A. Meyer. © 1999 John Wiley & Sons Ltd.

response is to consider if compliance and bioavailability have been adequate, and, if so, then to conclude that the patient's medical condition has deteriorated—prompting special maneuvers such as extraordinary diagnostic tests and therapeutic escalation in the form of higher doses and/or stronger agents. Without objective means to measure compliance or absorption, the prescribing physician is likely to fall back on what he or she knows best and conclude that worsening disease is the reason for inadequate response to the prescribed drug.

If the real explanation for failed treatment is poor compliance or poor bioavailability, however, then diagnostic and therapeutic maneuvers predicated on the false assumption of worsening disease are misdirected, their cost is basically needless, and the realization of any hazard that they pose only adds to the avoidable costs. In this scenario, poor bioavailability and poor compliance are functionally equivalent, though of course mechanistically dissimilar. Bioavailability problems have consistently received a great deal of professional and public attention, beginning with the bioavailability problems of digoxin in the early 1970s, continuing with the discovery and quantification of first-pass effects of various drugs, various food–drug and drug–drug interactions, and culminating most recently in the discovery of the wide array of mixed-function oxidases in the gut wall. Meanwhile, biopharmaceutics has attracted major research investment, many changes in pharmaceutical labeling, and various educational efforts to minimize variability in bioavailability. In contrast, the topic of patient compliance has been mostly ignored, although the prevalence of substandard drug exposure due to compliance problems is probably much greater than that due to problems of absorption or first-pass metabolism. The reasoning behind this assertion is that poor and partial compliance appear to affect *all* drugs used in ambulatory care, not just those with special biopharmaceutical characteristics. One key difference, of course, is that most compliance problems result in under- rather than overexposure to the drugs in question[1]. Thus, the clinical complications created by poor/partial compliance tend to mimic those of worsening disease, whereas biopharmaceutical problems often create overexposure and associated toxicity problems, which tend to have a characteristic clinical signature.

Any well-considered systems analysis of the sources of variance in drug response (e.g. that of Harter and Peck[2]) shows the need to balance the investments made in attack on the various sources when the aim is to improve the overall reliability of drug response. The medical and economic consequences of variable drug responses are a topic in their own right. Variable dosing due to variable compliance is, however, a leading contributor to overall variability in drug response, as assessed in groups of patients. Obviously individual patients who dose correctly—a modest majority—will be free of this source of variability in their responses, but the practical use of this fact in clinical decision-making requires reliable information on compliance.

The validity of the electronically compiled dosing history is subject to certain, relatively minor, limitations[1]. Other chapters in this book present the various findings of EM, which will not be repeated here except to reiterate the basic theme that the main expression of patient non-compliance is a recurring array of widely varying delays and omissions of regimen-specified doses. Extra doses are occasionally taken, and, while they may pose special problems for drugs with abuse potential or with especially narrow therapeutic indices, such errors of commission are about 25% as common as errors of omission[1]. This chapter thus focuses on the economic consequences of the more prevalent errors of omission in dosing.

A NOTE ON PHARMACOTHERAPEUTICS

Pharmacotherapeutics is a diverse body of knowledge about the actions of pharmaceuticals in humans, and the outcomes of their ongoing use. Given the diversity of human disease and the actions of the thousand or so agents that make up the active pharmacopoeia, there are relatively few generalizations, most of the information being specific to drug, formulation, disease, and comorbidity. This same consideration applies to the consequences of suboptimal treatment, of which non/poor/partial compliance are categories, although suboptimal treatment also includes the prescribing of a suboptimal regimen for a rationally selected drug, or the prescribing of an irrationally chosen drug. It is useful to begin with a consideration of the few generalizations that can serve as guides to understanding the therapeutic and economic implications of dosing that strays from the optimal.

Three Generalizations

One generalization is the dose–response relation, because dose-dependency of drug action is a fundamental property of all drugs.

Another generalization is the time-dependency of drug action, as all drug actions vary with time since the last dose taken, typically peaking more or less soon after dose administration then waning more or less gradually. The time dependencies of long-maintained sequences of dose administration are also a part of this story. In overview, one can say that the magnitude of the action of most drugs increases as dose increases, or as doses are held constant but clustered more closely together in time; also that drug actions wane with the passage of time since the last-taken dose—rapidly with some pharmaceuticals, more slowly with others, and (with some drugs) more rapidly early and less rapidly later in a long-maintained course of treatment.

A third generalization is that drug action is the outcome of interplay between pharmacological mechanisms and physiologic, homeostatic, counter-regulatory mechanisms. Each set of mechanisms will have its characteristic time course of onset of action/counteraction following drug administration, and of offset of action/counteraction once drug administration has ended.

Notes on Counter-regulatory Actions

When the pharmacologic mechanism begins much sooner than the counter-regulatory action, the initial doses will, in general, be smaller than those needed after the counter-regulatory mechanisms come into play. Starting with the eventual dose incurs the risk of overdose toxicity, so drugs with this attribute are referred to as having a 'first-dose effect', implying that the initial doses must be smaller than the eventual ones. First-dose effects are usually quickly discerned early in drug development, as it is soon discovered that the dose must be escalated in order to maintain a therapeutically useful drug response. Less obvious, but also important, is what happens long after the final dose level has been reached when a drug holiday occurs and dosing is interrupted for some days. If the no-dose interval is long enough for the counter-regulatory mechanisms to fade, then the resumption of dosing should follow the same sequence of escalation from an initially low dose at the outset of dosing. In actuality, however, drug holidays are almost invariably initiated by the patient, often unwittingly, and are rarely recognized clinically, and so a natural course of events is for dosing to be resumed at the accustomed full-strength level, with its accompanying risk of overdose toxicity. These are called 'recurrent first-dose effects', and have probably been responsible for the forced withdrawal of some otherwise useful agents from the pharmaceutical market[1].

If the counter-regulatory mechanism fades much more slowly than the pharmacologic action, the result of a sudden halt of dosing will be a period of unopposed, counter-regulatory action, which may result in some kind of rebound effect, in which the drug-regulated variable surges to levels more hazardous than those that prevailed before drug treatment was ever begun. An example of this sequence of events is seen with beta-adrenergic receptor blockers of the class that lack intrinsic sympathomimetic activity—the so-called 'non-ISA' beta-blockers, which include the ones most widely used: propranolol, atenolol, and metoprolol. The labeling for these agents includes warnings against sudden discontinuation of dosing, which is known to heighten the risk of incident coronary disease[3–5]. The counter-regulatory response to beta-receptor blockade is upregulation of beta-receptors; when beta-blocker dosing halts the receptors return to normal with a half-life of about a week[6]; in contrast the non-ISA beta-blockers have a half-life of less than half a day[6]. Thus, a sudden halt in dosing results in rapid disappearance of beta-receptor blockade, and gradual disappearance of exaggerated adrenergic responses to physiologically triggered sympathetic nerve activity or catecholamine secretion—two key consequences of which are increased platelet aggregation and vascular spasm, both substrates for incident coronary heart disease[4].

The interplay of primary pharmacologic actions and secondary physiologic counteractions is an underdeveloped topic in both basic pharmacology and drug development. Long considered a rather academic topic, this interplay assumes pragmatic importance in light of the incidence of drug holidays, which impose and reimpose sudden halts in dosing, variably long lapses in dosing, and sudden resumptions in dosing, usually at full strength. As a result, the drug holiday is coming to be seen as a novel source of toxicity—novel in two senses, because holidays were not recognized until recently[7], and because they represent toxicity from *under*dosing[8]. A further aspect of this topic concerns very slowly developing physiological responses to primary drug actions, resulting in very gradual changes in the drug's apparent pharmacodynamics—such that, for example, the offset of drug action when long-maintained dosing suddenly halts is much more gradual than seen when dosing is halted after only a few days or weeks of treatment. These very slow pharmacodynamic changes may allow rather radical decreases in daily dose requirements, which can have major economic implications, given that pharmaceutical pricing is dose-dependent, based on short-term dose–response characteristics, and (in most countries) fixed.

Overview

One byproduct of the electronic renaissance in compliance research has been a gradual recognition among clinical pharmacologists of the need to under-stand the consequences of the temporal patterns of dosing actually observed in relatively large numbers of patients. This new information has put the focus on a relatively neglected topic in clinical pharmacology: what happens when dosing suddenly stops, as it so often does in the course of ambulatory phar-macotherapy, in both trials and practice. The new focus on quantifying pa-tients' dosing histories has highlighted the need to know:

- how long drug action can persist at a therapeutically useful level when long-maintained dosing stops,
- whether drug-modulated physiologic variables tend to rebound to haz-ardous levels after dosing stops,
- whether dosing, once interrupted, can safely resume at the usual dosing level or must, to avoid 'first-dose' toxicity, be restarted at a lower level and gradually stepped upwards.

These aspects are considered in other chapters of this book, but are the salient aspects of the clinical pharmacodynamics that determine the clinical and econ-omic consequences of variable compliance. A direct consequence of having reli-able data on dosing histories is the ability to quantify discrepancies between prescribed and actual dosing. Indeed, the modern definition of drug regimen compliance is the extent to which the patient's dosing history conforms to the prescribed drug regimen[1]. This perspective naturally illuminates two further aspects of pharmacodynamics. One is the margin for errors in dose-timing that can occur without attenuation of the drug response elicited by correct, per-regimen dosing. This aspect is called 'forgiveness'[1]. The second aspect is whether the recommended regimen is optimal, or whether it calls for doses that are substantially higher or lower or are given more or less often, than necessary.

Historically, recommended regimens that later turned out to be suboptimal erred mainly on the side of overdosing[9]. Setting the dose at higher-than-necessary levels is one way to obtain forgiveness for, in general, the higher the dose the longer it takes for a drug's actions to wane to subtherapeutic levels, though the higher dose is also more likely to elicit undesirable side-effects.

As with many of the pharmacometric aspects of patient compliance, this point was first recognized in the field of oral contraception, after estrogen doses in oral contraceptives were reduced in the late 1960s in order to avoid the thrombogenic effects of the original, high-estrogen preparations. Lowering the estrogen dose minimized the thrombogenic effects but also substantially narrowed the limits of variability in dose timing consistent with full contraceptive efficacy[10,11]—a trade-off that may be expected to recur from time to time in other therapeutic situations.

ANALYZING THE ECONOMICS OF POOR OR PARTIAL COMPLIANCE

This topic logically breaks down into three parts. The first is to understand whether a dose not taken—the most common error of compliance—is also a dose not purchased. Obviously if a drug is being purchased but not taken, the costs of both treatment and untreated disease are incurred. The second is to consider what generalizations can be made about the clinical consequences of taking, relative to the recommended regimen, fewer doses, more widely separated in time, than called for. The third part is to translate those clinical consequences into economic terms.

In these considerations, there are substantial differences between acute-use and chronic-use pharmaceuticals, and, among the latter, between prophylactic and therapeutic applications.

IS A DOSE UNTAKEN A DOSE NOT PURCHASED?

This question may also be put as: 'does poor or partial compliance reduce the cost of acquiring drug?' A dose taken is a dose purchased, unless it is part of a sampling program. The answer to the inverse question, however, is more complex.

The continued purchasing of never-taken drug obviously adds to the costs of untreated disease. It is an extreme situation that may prevail for some time with some patients, but its indefinite continuation is probably exceptional for several reasons. First, poor compliers appear to have a higher likelihood of early discontinuation of even the pretense of treatment[12]; second, unused medicine accumulates and requires storage space, emphasizing the futility of purchasing never-used drug, even at a third party's expense. Nevertheless, the accumulation of untaken medicines can be formidable, as exemplified by a report that the Canadian Province of Alberta had collected 26 tonnes of unused pharmaceuticals in a special program that is repeated biennially in their population of approximately 2.5 million people[13]. This figure represents, with reasonable allowances for packaging materials, syringes, and other non-pharmaceutical materials that were probably included in this 'trashcan perspective', about 5 g of unused pharmaceutical per person, equivalent to several dozen tablets/capsules per person of all ages.

The more common case is the patient who some of the time takes the prescribed dose, and whose acquisition of drug is loosely coupled to actual consumption. The coupling has two models, the Anglo-Saxon and the Continental (discussed below). First a distinction must be drawn between acute-use and chronic-use medicines.

Acute-use Medicines

If the drug is prescribed for use during a single episode of illness, then its underuse will result in leftover drugs that may be available for a subsequent episode of illness. This carries the potential for inappropriate self-prescribing and for use of outdated product.

Chronic-use Medicines

Long-term pharmacotherapy is based on sequential prescriptions written for usually 1–3 months' supply. The specific duration is determined by the cost of the pharmaceutical and factors of custom and convenience. The process by which the patient obtains a renewed supply of medicine differs considerably between the Anglo-Saxon (USA, Canada, UK) and the Continental (France, Germany and other European) countries.

Anglo-Saxon Policy

In the Anglo-Saxon countries, once it is apparent that the patient is tolerating the medicine and responding suitably to the selected dose, the physician will usually write a prescription allowing for multiple refills, which puts the timing of prescription refills at the patient's discretion, driven, usually, by imminent exhaustion of the patient's supply of drug. Return visits to the physician, for routine follow-up, are not linked to the refilling of the prescription, and will occur at intervals set by custom, policy, economics, and convenience. If the patient complies poorly or partially with the prescribed regimen, he or she will take longer to exhaust the supply of drug and tend, therefore, to postpone the time when the prescription is refilled, although the schedule of return visits to the physician will continue at its own rate. In some patients, a tendency to poor compliance with the drug regimen may also be associated with missing scheduled return appointments[14].

The net effect of the Anglo-Saxon refill policy is to create a strong link between consumption and purchasing. The residual quantity of drug from the prior prescription may vary when the next refill is sought, making the correlation between aggregate drug intake and prescription refill interval somewhat variable, but this source of variability shrinks as the observation period lengthens. This, and other considerations in using refill intervals as a measure of aggregate drug intake, have been discussed by Steiner and colleagues[15].

Continental Policy

In contrast, the Continental system of prescribing is based on the use of the so-called 'original pack'—in general, a 4-week supply of solid dosage forms in a calendar-type of unit-dose 'blister' package. The next follow-up visit is scheduled for the time when the patient's last-dispensed supply of drug would be exhausted, assuming full compliance with the prescribed regimen. At the next visit the physician gives the patient a new prescription to replenish the (presumably dwindled) supply of drug, thus allowing treatment to continue. If the patient has complied poorly or partially, the supply will have dwindled only partly, but that fact is not often revealed to the physician. It appears to be a common occurrence that poorly/partially compliant patients convey to their physicians the impression that they dose correctly. The upshot of this is that the new prescription is usually written although the patient may or may not have it filled. Such factors as copayment, reimbursement, recollection of the supply of unused medicine, and psychological pressures from prescriber or pharmacist appear to influence the patient's decision to fill the prescription.

The interval between follow-up visits differs between countries: it tends to be monthly in countries that pay physicians by the visit, quarterly in countries that pay physicians an annual capitation fee.

Does the Interval Between Visits Matter?

Whether the interval between visits has appreciable influence on patient compliance is an area for research. Two pieces of evidence are noteworthy.

One is the finding by Wasson *et al.* of a 29% reduction in aggregate health resource consumption when the frequency of contact between physician and patient was increased by the use of between-visit phone calls by the physician[16]. This finding, confirmed in a randomized, controlled trial, is both startling and challenging. The underlying mechanism(s) were not defined by the study, but it is probable that more frequent contact makes it possible to identify and resolve early certain problems that would be more difficult and costly to resolve if not discovered until later.

The second noteworthy finding is that some poor or partial compliers improve their compliance around the time of scheduled follow-up visits[17,18]. Alvan Feinstein named this effect 'white-coat compliance'[19]: it appears to be limited to 2–3 days on either side of the visit. The effect probably contributes less to therapeutic benefit than to diagnostic confusion, because it tends to drive drug-influenced clinical observables into desirable ranges (as Feinstein noted), favoring the clinical impression that the patient is being treated effectively. Discrepancies arise when a relatively rapidly drug-responsive surrogate marker, such as blood pressure or intraocular pressure, is well controlled at successive office visits while slow-to-change structural indices of disease (e.g. persistent left ventricular hypertrophy in hypertension or ongoing optic nerve damage in glaucoma—neither of which could be expected to respond to a few days per month of correct treatment), which reflect the usually prevailing situation, remain in a pathological range. A usually overlooked aspect of white-coat compliance is that its occurrence signifies that patients can and do respond with correct compliance when they see, or think they see, medical attention being directed toward the quality of their execution of agreed-upon drug regimens.

It is likely that the length of the interval between visits has a modest effect on aggregate consumption of drug, as the following simulation suggests.

> A patient who persistently omits, on average, one dose in three is seen monthly; the patient complies fully during the 3 days before the visit, the day of the visit, and the 3 days following. His aggregate consumption of drug will be 14 once-daily tablets in the three 'non-visit' weeks, and seven tablets during the 'visit' week. The aggregate 4-weekly intake of drug would be 21 tablets, or 75% of prescribed doses taken, vs the running rate, without white-coat compliance, of 67%. In contrast, if the same patient were seen at 12-week intervals, the white-coat effect would operate only once instead of three times, with an average monthly intake of drug of 77×0.67 during the 11 'non-visit' weeks, plus seven doses during the 'visit' week. So a total of 59 doses would be taken: 59/84 (= 70%) of prescribed doses taken.

Such differences in drug consumption are small and probably have only incidental medical importance, but they do signify a potentially important point in the context of the large sums of promotional money spent in the quest for a few percentage point gains in market share. After all, a 5% increase in consumption by patients prescribed a product with a 20% market share would, in the Anglo-Saxon refill policy, produce a one-point gain in share. Yet to gain a one-point share of a competitive market by conventional means entails a promotional barrage that typically invites competitive counterbarrages, echoing the trench warfare of World War I, with both sides expending vast resources with little or no net gain. The same money might yield greater increases in product sales when invested in means to bring more patients into optimal consumption of pharmaceuticals already prescribed.

Irrespective of the effects, if any, of the frequency of physician visits the net effect of the Continental system appears to be to drive chronic-use pharmaceutical acquisition costs closer to the full-compliance level than in the Anglo-Saxon system. However, the specific, quantitative aspects of this difference remain to be studied. One may wonder if either system especially favors good compliance, but no studies appear to have been undertaken on the point. The range of compliance is equally wide under the two systems, indicating that neither is ideal, regardless of modest differences in mean or median compliance.

The foregoing underscores the fact that much is to be learned about how to optimize the provision of health services.

Economic Implications for Refilling Prescriptions for Chronic-use Medicines

As average consumption rates tend to run in the range of 80–85%, there is a potential diminution in refill rates, and thus product sales, of something on the order of 15–20% of the annual turnover for chronic-use, ambulatory-care pharmaceuticals. However, averages often mislead, and so it is useful to look at the frequency histogram of deviations from the ideal in each situation, with the aim of targeting patients well below the mean or median, some of whom probably could, with a few simple steps, dramatically improve their compliance. In terms of increased sales of chronic-use, high-margin pharmaceuticals, a US$50–100 expenditure per properly targeted patient may be cost-effective.

Variations

Several firms in the USA have devised programs that urge patients to refill their prescriptions for chronic-use medicines at the time predicted by the assumption of full compliance. (The time interval between dispensing and refilling, called the 'legend duration', is calculated by dividing the number of tablets dispensed by the daily number of tablets to be taken[20].) It is doubtful whether such programs achieve substantive increases in actual drug consumption, or merely succeed in filling the patient's medicine cabinet, increasing the amounts of drug sold, and driving up someone's pharmaceutical expenditures without offsetting benefits.

Summing Up

The whole area of national and regional differences in the timing of doctor–patient and pharmacist–patient interactions is ripe for careful study, as exemplified by the remarkable results of Wasson et al.[16]. The consequences of variable compliance with prescribed drug regimens is a part of this story but was not an aspect that Wasson considered. It is, however, evident that suboptimal compliance with the regimens for crucial drugs can, when clinically unrecognized as such, have consequences that masquerade as worsened disease and create diagnostic confusion, as discussed earlier.

An early indicator of the value of positively identifying patients who are systematically non-compliant are the findings of Schneider and her colleagues[21]. They routinely use electronic monitoring of compliance as the first step in workup of patients referred with a diagnosis of drug-refractory hypertension: preliminary findings are that 30% of such patients are systematically non-compliant, not unresponsive, to drugs[21]. The economics of this will be discussed later.

SPECIFIC EXAMPLES

A widely used application of chronic pharmacotherapy is risk reduction in people presently without overt pathology—reducing the probability of future occurrence of one or more adverse events or conditions. For example, the aim of treating people with anatomically normal cardiovascular systems who have mild or moderate hypertension is to reduce the probabilities of a debilitating stroke and of developing coronary heart disease (CHD), with its various sequelae (which include myocardial revascularization procedures such as coronary bypass surgery or angioplasty, myocardial infarction), or congestive heart failure, with its sequelae of pathological fluid retention, serious cardiac arrhythmias, dyspnea, curtailed mobility, and death. The aim of treating the hyperlipidemias is to reduce the probability of coronary heart disease and its sequelae. The aim of various hormonal and mineral regimens in peri- and post-menopausal women is to prevent osteoporosis, and its consequent fractures, deformities, pain, and impaired mobility. The list of chronic diseases for which prophylactic treatment is available grows, but the notion of chronic administration of drugs for purely preventive purposes in otherwise healthy people is less than 40 years old, beginning with oral contraception.

Common to these treatment regimens is the aim of risk reduction—to reduce the likelihood of consequences which create overt pathology, impair the quality of life, and increase the risk of death.

Note on Probability, Likelihood, Risk

The terms 'likelihood' and 'risk' are used interchangeably here. In the present context they have identical meanings, with 'risk' carrying the more narrow implication of 'the likelihood of something bad happening'[22]. Thus, one would not normally speak of the 'risk of benefit', though one could equally correctly speak of the 'likelihood of benefit' or the 'likelihood of harm'. With this qualification, the proper usage of all three terms requires two specifications:

1. The phenomenon whose likelihood of future occurrence is at issue.
2. The time period within which we tabulate occurrence or non-occurrence of the phenomenon in question.

Note on Treatment vs Prophylaxis, and Primary vs Secondary Prevention

It may seem more apt to describe some pharmaceutical regimens as 'prophylaxis' rather than 'treatment', although the distinction is blurred by the fact that the underlying diseases tend to have long-running subclinical antecedents. CHD, for example, is often an incidental finding at autopsy of relatively young men who died of unrelated causes. The walls of major arteries contained clinically unsuspected atheromatous plaques, which were presumably destined, had not death for other reasons intervened, to declare themselves clinically after they had become sufficiently severe to critically reduce blood flow through a major coronary artery. Thus, with expanded knowledge of the natural history of disease, the boundary between prophylaxis and treatment shifts to an earlier point in the disease process, blurring a once-sharp boundary.

Some draw the distinction between primary and secondary prevention, the former being reserved for patients who have none of the presently accepted clinical criteria of disease (e.g. no angina, previous myocardial infarction, congestive heart failure, arrhythmias, or history or diagnostic manifestations of any). Still, an overweight 63-year-old man with elevated cholesterol levels but no other symptoms could have quite extensive arterial atheromatous lesions, which would be evident only if coronary angiography were included in routine clinical diagnostic procedures. Thus, a change in diagnostic practice can also move the boundary between 'primary' and 'secondary' prevention, as well as between 'prophylaxis' and 'treatment'. Such a change could be catalyzed by a methodologic advance that (for example) permitted visualization of the patterns of blood flow in coronary arteries without the present need to catheterize the coronary arteries, thus reserving the procedure for patients with overt manifestations of CHD.

Although the boundary between primary and secondary prevention studies can be 'fuzzy' in the earlier stages of disease, there is an important difference, which is accentuated by variable patient compliance.

Important Distinction Between Primary and Secondary Prevention Studies

As disease worsens, the need generally grows for multiple medications. The situation is well illustrated by CHD, the use of which as an example is reinforced by its being both widely prevalent and a leading cause of death. As CHD progresses to the point at which congestive heart failure develops, the patient's homeostatic mechanisms lose their normal ability to maintain salt and water balance, and the patient begins to retain some or all of their daily dietary salt intake. The mechanisms of osmolar homeostasis remain intact, and insure that retention of salt is accompanied by retention of sufficient water to maintain isotonicity (about 1 liter for each 150 mmol (8.8 g) of salt retained). As heart failure worsens, retention of dietary salt approaches completeness and, concomitantly, the ability of the failing cardiovascular system to accommodate extra fluid diminishes, putting the untreated patient on a collision course with the sequence of salt retention leading to water retention, leading to peripheral edema, leading to pulmonary venous congestion, leading to acute pulmonary edema, with its high risk of death. A crucial pharmacotherapeutic step is therefore the use of a natriuretic agent such as furosemide that can restore the normal equality between salt excretion and intake. A patient has been cited with moderate to severe congestive heart failure who skipped three days of prescribed furosemide, saving about $0.15 in drug costs. However, she then developed acute pulmonary congestion and spent 6 days in hospital, for a cost of almost US$10 000[23].

Supporting care includes use of cardiotonic agents such as digoxin or digitoxin, beta-adrenergic receptor blockers, and agents that block the production or the actions of angiotensin II. The role of supporting pharmacotherapy is to maintain as good cardiovascular function as possible, given the underlying myocardial pathology. While these supportive agents could be used suboptimally in many instances, it is probably the natriuretic agent that affords the least tolerance for suboptimal dosing because such errors translate directly into failure of salt excretion and retention of salt and water. Overdosing with a natriuretic is counteracted by strong homeostatic mechanisms that prevent critical depletion of extracellular fluid; skipping doses of diuretic allows salt and water retention against a short-term limit of about 2 liters before pulmonary venous congestion occurs. Thus, the pathophysiologic situation is forgiving of overdosing but unforgiving of underdosing. Small accumulations of salt can gradually cause many liters of pathological fluid accumulation, as tissues stretch to accommodate the extra fluid acquired in small increments. When tissues are taut, a sudden accumulation of several liters of fluid within a period of several days can be expected to tip the patient into acute pulmonary congestion, with progressively worsening dyspnea and incipient or actual pulmonary edema, which is a medical emergency with a high risk of death.

Against this background, the conduct of any single-agent trial in patients with congestive heart failure grows steadily more complex as heart failure worsens[24,25]. The effects of the trial agent have to be seen against the 'baseline' created by the dose-dependent actions of all the non-trial agents that are deemed essential to the patient's well-being. It is in this setting that variable compliance becomes an especially pressing issue for, as Cramer has recently shown[26], compliance with multiple agents prescribed for synchronous administration is tightly linked, omission of a dose of one agent being very likely to be accompanied by omission of other concomitantly prescribed agents.

One consequence of this tight coupling is the appearance of a 'pharmacoillusion', in the form of a big 'effect' of measured compliance with trial placebo, appearing in the analysis of the clinical correlates of compliance with the trial agent and its placebo. Several such instances have been reported[27,28], the first of which is frequently cited as 'evidence' that measured compliance has no role in the analysis of randomized controlled trials[29-32]. The instances of this effect are limited to secondary prevention trials, where non-trial medications are the rule rather than the exception, unlike primary prevention trials where non-trial medications are exceptional and (when used) are rarely crucial for the patient's well-being. Thus, the probable pharmacologic consequences of suboptimal use of powerful, concomitantly prescribed non-trial medicines account for the 'effect' of variable compliance with trial placebo[25] rather than, as postulated in the re-analysis of the Coronary Drug Trial[27], mysterious 'lifestyle' factors so powerful as to make a 40% difference in mortality between good and poor compliers.

A much less convoluted and thus more plausible explanation is the array of the pharmacologic consequences of erratic compliance with non-trial agents, for which placebo compliance is only a proxy or surrogate measure, but it is a topic for research not polemic. Careful meta-analysis and other focused research is needed to ascertain whether the correlates of variable compliance with placebo appear in primary as well as secondary prevention trials because it is only in the latter that the 'effects' of placebo compliance can have a pharmacologic basis.

Almost two decades have passed since the re-analysis of the CDP trial was published, showing what (until very recently) was the biggest 'effect' ever seen in any trial on means to prevent CHD. In that time the clinical trialists and their acolytes have repeatedly invoked the CDP trial results to support the case for intention-to-treat (ITT) analysis, together with repeated cautions in favor of ignoring actual patterns of drug exposure in controlled clinical trials. Recently, both David Cox and Bradley Efron have called for the replacement of ITT analysis by systematic measurement of drug exposure in ambulatory trials and careful analysis to understand the clinical correlation of variable exposure[33,34]. Hasford[35], Feinstein[36], Efron[37], and Sheiner and Rubin[38] have also made this point.

Note on Relative vs Absolute Risk

Many clinical studies that compare the probabilities of occurrence of adverse outcomes do so in terms of relative risk reduction. A notable example is the Lipid Research Clinics Coronary Primary Prevention Trial (LRC-CPPT), the first trial to demonstrate that cholesterol reduction could reduce 'coronary risk'[39]. LRC-CPPT randomized 3906 patients to receive drug (24 g of cholestyramine, in three divided doses, or 4 g packets given in three divided doses) and placebo. Trial participants had to meet strict criteria for elevated concentrations of cholesterol in plasma, were free of the usual clinical signs/symptoms of CHD, and had little or no cholesterol-lowering response to a low-cholesterol diet (over 300 000 patients were screened to find the 3906 who actually participated in the study). After 7.2 years, 8.6% of the patients in the control group, compared with 7.0% in the group receiving cholestyramine, had developed one or more manifestations of CHD, a difference in absolute risk of coronary heart disease over the period of 1.6% that was deemed statistically significant ($p<0.05$; one-tailed t-test). This conclusion was controversial at the time[32], but its correctness has been repeatedly confirmed by many subsequent trials of other, stronger, lipid-lowering agents. The absolute risk reduction of 1.6% over 7.2 years can be annualized to 0.22% per year, a maneuver justified by the essential constancy of the drug effect during the trial[39].

Another way to represent the data is as relative risk reduction. The treatment reduced the relative risk of coronary heart disease by $100(8.6-7.0)/8.6 = 19\%$. The relative risk figure is a much larger, and thus more 'journalistic' number, than either of the absolute risks or their difference.

The Unicohort—Absolute Risk Translated to Facilitate Analysis and Communication

Another useful and informative way to express data is to consider how many patients must be treated in order to prevent one 'coronary event' per year. In the trial discussed above[39] the annualized reduction in absolute risk of developing CHD was 0.22%, which says that we must treat, on average, $100/0.22$ (= 450) patients for one year to prevent one patient from developing CHD.

This figure is conveniently called the 'unicohort'[22] because it is the size of the group needed to produce, on average, one beneficiary in the stated time period (here taken to be 1 year). It reflects the all-patient ITT average result associated with an average intake of drug that was slightly under half of the prescribed dose.

Economic Interpretation of the Unicohort

To treat 450 patients for one year has, within limits, a definable cost. The limits are set by the range of the amounts of drug purchased, which can be expected to vary between the amount taken by the patient (the limit under the Anglo-Saxon policy for prescribing-dispensing), and the full-compliance amount (the limit under the Continental policy). We can reckon these two limits, using the present average US wholesale price of cholestyramine of US\$39.3 per 4 g packet, which corresponds to US\$861 per year if all pre-scribed doses are purchased. The level of compliance associated with the all-patient average risk reduction was slightly less than half the prescribed dose of six packets per day: 2.7 packets per day. Thus, the cost of drug consumed under the Anglo-Saxon policy would be 2.7 × 365 × \$0.393 = \$387 per year. Treating 450 patients for one year will therefore cost between \$174 150 and the full-purchase cost of \$387 450, depending on the strength of the link between consumption and acquisition.

How Much is Saved by Preventing One Coronary Event?

These figures can be balanced against the cost of caring for a prevented 'coronary event', which can range from the almost zero cost of sudden death to a series of revascularization procedures (angioplasties of various kinds or coronary bypass). One of my patients, for example, needed three rather rapidly restenosed angioplasties followed by a multivessel bypass procedure for a total cost, at present levels, of about \$110 000, which is at the high end of care costs for coronary events that are not complicated by (for example) stroke, pulmonary embolus, or pneumonia. Present levels of reimbursement in the USA for treatment of a myocardial infarction range between \$12 000 and \$20 000, depending on complications, need for angioplasty, and other factors (based on US Diagnosis Related Groups 112, 116, 121, and 122). Thus, to calculate a 'typical' cost of prevention of a cardiac event one would have to construct, in the manner of the economic 'marketbasket', an incidence-weighted sum of costs of caring for the various sequelae of CHD.

Economic Consequences of Variable Compliance on Unicohort Size

The role of variable compliance can be seen from the virtually linear relation between average intake of cholestyramine and coronary risk reduction, together with a strong parallelism between relative cholesterol reduction and coronary risk reduction:

- 6.5% reduction in relative risk of CHD per 4-g packet consumed, averaged over the 5-year period of the study;
- 3.25% reduction in cholesterol levels per 4-g packet of drug consumed, averaged over the 5-year period of the study;
- 2% reduction in coronary risk for every 1% reduction in cholesterol levels.

The result of these unusually linear dose-dependent effects is that the unicohort sizes for avoiding one coronary event per year call for cholestyramine treatment of:

- 210 full compliers (six 4-g packets per day);
- 450 average compliers (2.7 packets per day);
- 757 bottom quartile compliers (1.5 packets per day).

The full-dose treatment cost for cholestyramine, using average US wholesale prices in 1996, was $861, so the cost of treating the unicohort of full compliers was US$180 800. In partially compliant patients, the two modes of prescribing-dispensing differed greatly in cost. In the Anglo-Saxon mode, the unicohort of bottom quartile patients cost approximately US$163 000— slightly less than predicted by a strictly linear dose–response relation because of a slight non-linearity in the compliance–effect curve in that region. The corresponding costs under the Continental mode were US$652 000. For average compliers, the Anglo-Saxon mode cost US$177 000, the Continental model estimate being US$387 000.

These comparisons demonstrate the potentially high cost of pushing refill prescriptions at clinically unrecognized poor and partial compliers. Another noteworthy point is that the almost linear relation between dose and effect cause both dose and effect to rise or fall together, keeping the cost of treating nearly unicohorts of widely differing sizes the same—provided that consumption and purchasing are tightly linked. Note, however, that the virtually linear relation between dose and effect of cholestyramine is exceptional. The more usual shape of dose–effect relations is hyperbolic, with three distinct regions:

- a low-dose region, within which changes in dose have little or no effect on drug response;
- an intermediate-dose region, within which relatively small changes in dose have a big effect on drug response;
- a high-dose region, within which changes in dose have little or no effect on drug response.

These hyperbolic relations may be linearized by using the logarithm of dose but, since medical practice involves actual rather than logarithmic doses, it is best to draw these relations arithmetically, as they prevail in practice. Later in this chapter we shall consider the case of gemfibrozil, another lipid-lowering agent with a typically hyperbolic relationship between dose and effect.

In contrast to the strong compliance-dependent effects in the drug-treated group, the placebo group showed no discernible effect of compliance on either coronary risk or lipid fractions. However, the range and distribution of compliance did differ between the two groups; a downward shift in compliance (by some 15% of prescribed doses) was noted in the active group compared with the placebo group[39]. This difference was probably related, in whole or in part, to the drug's dose-dependent impact on colonic gas generation, which leads patients occasionally to reduce the dose at times to minimize this action.

The More Representative Example of Gemfibrozil

The Helsinki Heart Study (HHS) of gemfibrozil was initiated several years after the LRC-CPPT began, and was published in the late 1980s[40]. The non-linear dose–effect relation of gemfibrozil is more typical of most drugs than the nearly linear one of cholestyramine. This difference means that the economic consequences of poor/partial compliance with the regimen for gemfibrozil are correspondingly larger.

The HHS Results

The 5-year absolute risk of coronary events was 4.1% in the placebo-treated group and 2.7% in the gemfibrozil-treated group[40]—corresponding to a relative risk reduction, by intention-to-treat analysis, of 34%. A more conservative estimate comes from a Cox proportional hazards model for drug action, in which benefit is solely attributed to the drug's dual effect—rise in HDL cholesterol and fall in LDL cholesterol, with coefficients for relative risk reduction of 0.029 and 0.015, respectively, for HDL rise and for LDL fall. Together these coefficients predict a 28% reduction on relative coronary risk for average compliers who took, in total, 84% of the prescribed dose.

The Cox model offered by the HHS analysts predicts relative risk reduction in the four quartiles of compliance as shown in Table 9.1.

It can be seen that the prophylactic effect of the drug fell by 72% as drug intake declined into the lowest quartile. In contrast, the placebo group showed no discernible effect of compliance on either coronary risk or lipid fractions[40]; moreover, the range and distribution of compliance were essentially identical in recipients of drug and of placebo. These findings support

TABLE 9.1   Relative risk reduction in the HHS[39]

Quartile of compliance	Percentage of doses taken	Predicted reduction in coronary risk (as percentage of placebo control)
4	>93	48.7
3	85–93	41.7
2	69–85	27.8
1	<69	13.9

the conclusion that the correlates of drug exposure in the drug group are a reflection of dose-dependent drug action, not of some hidden factor linked somehow to dosing behavior.

These compliance-dependent figures translate into the following unicohort sizes for drug-induced prevention of one case of incident CHD per year:

- 205 for the top quartile;
- 357 for the average complier;
- 719 for the bottom quartile.

The respective treatment costs are $205 \times \$723 = \$148\ 215$ for the top quartile The cost figure is the recent average wholesale price of a 1-year supply of gemfibrozil in the US market, fully complied with. In the Anglo Saxon purchas ing mode, the costs of treating the unicohort of average compliers is projected at $357 \times \$607 = \$216\ 700$, compared with $\$258\ 110$ in the Continental, full-acquisition mode. The costs of treating the unicohort of fourth-quartile compliers is $719 \times$ about $\$362 = $ ca. $\$260\ 278$ in the Anglo-Saxon mode and $\$519\ 837$ in the Continental, full-acquisition mode. The high cost of treating the fourth quartile reflects the non-linearity in the dose–response relation for gemfibrozil, and the fact that the lowest quartile patients prescribed gemfibrozil appeared to be taking a much larger fraction of the prescribed dose than were the lowest quartile of patients prescribed cholestyramine.

Conclusions from LRC-CPPT and HHS

These two primary prevention trials against CHD have striking similarities and dissimilarities. The unicohort sizes in the two trials were similar, despite the marked differences in physical aspects of the two dosing regimens and modes of action. The economic correlates in the Continental, full-acquisition mode of prescribing-dispensing show a similar inflation in costs when large numbers of patients purchase large amounts of drug, the benefits of which are lost because little drug is actually taken. When purchasing is linked to actual use, in the Anglo-Saxon mode, the key factor becomes the shape of the compliance–effect relationship. The near-linearity of that relationship for cholestyramine almost neutralizes the economic impact of poor/partial compliance because benefits and costs change together. In contrast, the more typically hyperbolic shape of the exposure–effect relationship found in the compliance-stratification of HHS includes a region wherein the relationship declines steeply, so that patients in the fourth quartile are purchasing substantial amounts of drug but getting little or no benefit. This last point is an economic variation on a theme, described by Levy in pharmacological terms[41].

These points are illustrated by three variants in dose-response relation (Figures 9.1–9.3). Comparison of the three figures shows how drugs with similar actions but dissimilar dose–response relationships can be more or less forgiving of lapses in dosing.

Figures 9.1–9.3 illustrate how changes in the shape of the dose–response relation (or cost–benefit relation, in economic terms) can influence the economic impact of poor/partial compliance. The zone of forgiveness allows dosage and acquisition cost to fall with little or no impact on beneficial action. If the drug developer opts to revise the recommended dose down toward the point where the curve starts to break, the maneuver will eliminate the margin for error when medication is omitted or delayed, and will dilute estimates of efficacy in intention-to-treat analyses of any trials that may be run with the no-forgiveness regimen. If a cost-conscious managed care organization decides to eliminate the zone of forgiveness by lowering the recommended dose, drug acquisition costs will be lower but extra costs will be incurred to treat unavoided coronary events—and potentially bad publicity when its cost-cutting maneuvers come to light.

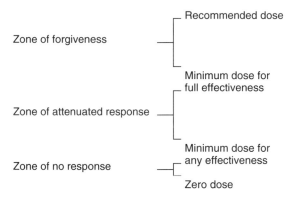

FIGURE 9.1 Ideal dose–response relation, in which the recommended dose is separated by some distance from the minimum dose needed for full effectiveness, creating a moderately-sized 'zone of forgiveness' within which dosing can vary with little or no attenuation of benefit—a safety margin, in other words. Below lies a 'zone of attenuated response', within which response declines as dosing declines, not necessarily proportionally but, in some instances, with marked disproportion such that a small decline in dose produces a large decline in response. Below the zone of attenuated response is a 'zone of no response', within which dosing may vary but without evident response

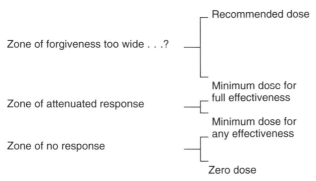

FIGURE 9.2 Dose–response relation in which the 'zone of forgiveness' is unusually wide, perhaps too wide, in allowing dosing to be reduced by a substantial fraction without any discernible impact on the drug response, and tempting would-be cost-cutters to tinker with the recommended dosing regimen. Below the minimum dose for full effectiveness, however, the response falls off very steeply to zero, with a small zone within which dose can vary without evident response

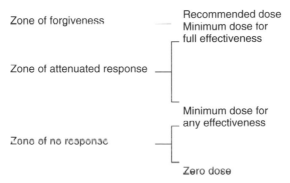

FIGURE 9.3 A drug with a very small zone of forgiveness such that small decreases in dose, below the recommended level, result in substantial reductions in drug response. The zone of attenuated response is in this example relatively wide; it could be considerably narrower. The remainder of the relation is unremarkable

Overview of Prophylactic Treatment

A notable aspect of prophylactic treatment is that 'treatment failure' is essentially undefinable at the level of the individual patient. In primary prevention, as we have seen, several hundred patients must be treated for a year to prevent a single occurrence of the targeted condition; moreover, the incidence of the target condition is lower (but not zero) in the treated group. One form of treatment failure is, however, recognizable at the level of the individual patient: the occurrence of some kind of adverse reaction to the prophylactic agent(s), e.g. the rare case of rhabdomyolysis with gemfibrozil or the statin group of cholesterol-lowering agents. Other more commonly occurring side-effects (e.g. the various gastrointestinal side-effects of cholestyramine) appear to be dose-dependent. Thus the individual patient can develop a more or less clear view of the drug's dose-dependent costs and side-effects, but no perception of the benefits, which are defined actuarially and presented in drug labeling. When benefits are based solely on ITT averages they are diluted, giving the compliant majority a substantial underestimate of the beneficial consequences of taking the drug correctly. As Lasagna and Hutt have pointed out[42], this type of misinformation is technically a form of mislabeling, for it is a point at which the ethical principle of full-disclosure labeling conflicts with the statistical principle of ITT analysis. The solution to this problem, as David Cox has recently pointed out, is to perform several different analyses, at least one of which takes into account the estimated effects of variable dosing[33].

EXPRESSING THE BENEFITS OF CHRONIC-USE DRUG REGIMENS FOR TREATMENT OF PATHOLOGICAL PROCESSES

We now turn to another class of agent; those that play a direct role in the management or control or suppression of pathological processes. In general, the effectiveness of these agents can be judged in individual patients because every patient in this category is ill with one or more conditions that require ongoing treatment in order to normalize (or at least beneficially modulate) the patient's condition. Examples of treatment failure are listed in Table 9.2.

TABLE 9.2   Examples of failed pharmacotherapy

Seizures during treatment with antiepileptic drugs
Persistent or episodic hypertension during treatment with antihypertensive agents
Hyperglycemia and rise in glycosylated hemoglobin during treatment with hypoglycemic agents
Relapse, recurrence, and/or emergence of drug-resistant microorganisms during treatment with anti-infective agents
Acute fluid retention during treatment of congestive heart failure
Life-threatening arrhythmias during treatment with antiarrhythmic agents
Thromboembolic phenomena during treatment with anticoagulants
Flare-up of inflammatory disease during treatment with anti-inflammatory agents
Acute rejection of a transplanted organ during treatment with immunosuppressants
Relapse of depression during treatment with an antidepressant
Conception during treatment with ovulation-inhibiting steroids
Acute exacerbations of asthma during antiasthma treatment

Note the great diversity of events that define failed pharmacotherapy: for this reason, it is difficult to draw more than two major generalizations about this array of situations.

> Generalization 1: The consequences of total or substantial non-compliance with a rationally prescribed regimen of an effective agent will, in general, mimic the worsening of disease and/or drug-refractory disease.

Thus, lurking in every case of failed pharmacotherapy is, as noted before, the diagnostic riddle: pharmacological non-response or non-compliance? Clinicians frequently overestimate patient compliance, or otherwise fail to recognize it when non-compliance is the root cause of what appears to be either worsening disease or drug non-responsiveness. This setting is one in which a few weeks' use of an electronic monitor to ascertain the actual patterns of dosing can be valuable.

This conclusion is underscored by the studies of Schneider and her colleagues in Lausanne on 'drug refractory hypertension'. In their region it is the policy for general practitioners to use a stepped-care scheme to treat newly diagnosed hypertensive patients. If a patient progresses through several steps of escalated treatment without discernible lowering of blood pressure, he or she is referred to the University Hospital for diagnostic work-up. Formerly, such patients would be worked up in a sequence of tests that cost about SFr2000 but during 1997 this center changed its policy, and now starts each referred patient on a 2-month period of electronic monitoring of compliance with a basic, single-agent, antihypertensive regimen. This maneuver reveals that one patient in about three is systematically non-compliant[21]. The cost of this monitoring study is about SFr200 per patient, although it will probably decline in the future as monitor usage increases. Despite the presently relatively high cost, however, the monitoring of three patients (at a cost of SFr600) avoids one diagnostic work-up costing SFr2000 and avoids the risks the work-up incurs, of which the greatest comes from the renal angiogram that is part of the work-up of truly drug refractory hypertension.

> Generalization 2: One-fifth of the patients create four-fifths of the cost.

'Cost' is synonymous with caregiver time, tests, difficulties, and money spent. This generalization is obviously not to be taken literally, but as an approximate 'rule of thumb'. A practical way to put this generalization on a quantitative footing in a specific situation is to adopt a form of analysis that I term 'suttonomic analysis'[43], after the famous bank-robber Willie Sutton who, after having been jailed several times for bank robbery, was asked why he robbed banks. 'Because', he said, 'that's where the money is.' Suttonomic analysis thus defines 'where the money is', or perhaps more aptly 'was', because it rank-orders patients with a particular disease problem by either the aggregate costs of their care, or some other measure of resource utilization during a previous period of apt duration (e.g. a year). A markedly skewed frequency histogram, in which about four-fifths of costs are clustered among one-fifth of the patients, would be expected.

Those high-cost patients are the natural target for focused investigation, which should include quantitative measurements of compliance with the regimen that is crucial to their effective care. The design of such investigations is a challenge, not the least because it is (or should be) a patient-specific effort to identify the trigger for a period of high-cost treatment and will almost invariably entail hospitalization.

Useful examples are the several recently published results of telephone intervention programs in the management of patients with moderate to severe congestive heart failure[44,45]. In these studies, patients with a record of costly complications are put in touch with a specially trained individual, usually a nurse, who several times a week talks with the patient, probing for evidence of fluid retention or other incipient complications of congestive heart failure and institutes early intervention to prevent worsening. None of these programs has to date used objective measures of drug regimen compliance but, with the clinical focus sharply on the search for incipient failure of treatment in patients at high risk of same, compliance monitoring may not be essential for cost-effective management. As experience grows with these new techniques, and as costs of monitoring key clinical variables decline, telephone intervention programs can be expected to seek the greatest cost-efficiency. Achieving that goal may involve ongoing monitoring of patients' drug regimen compliance, if indeed errors in compliance are commonly involved in exacerbations of the disease, and if early warning of missed doses improves the efficiency of disease management.

CONCLUDING OVERVIEW

The diversity of human diseases—about 1000 items in the ICD—and the comparable diversity of pharmacologic agents available for their prevention, mitigation, or cure—about 1000 substances in the active pharmacopoeia—creates a formidable array of qualitatively and quantitatively different therapeutic situations. Even further diversity arises when the dimension of variable patient compliance with prescribed drug regimens is added, not only because of the diverse dosing patterns that occur but also because some recommended regimens are suboptimal to begin with, and recommended drug regimens differ widely in their degrees of forgiveness for patterns of dosing other than the one(s) recommended.

Case-by-case analysis is thus inescapable, guided by only a few generalizations. Two basic generalizations are that drug actions depend on the quantity of drug taken at each dose, and on the time intervals between doses. Noncompliance, poor compliance, and partial compliance mean less drug taken, at longer intervals, than deemed optimal—the 'deeming' having been done on various grounds ranging from sound science to raw guessing, heavily seasoned with pharmacokinetic data (ab)used as a surrogate for pharmacodynamic response times.

On the economic side, less drug taken more often than not (though not always) means less money spent on purchasing the drug. Suboptimal treatment incurs the likelihood, but usually not the certainty, of suboptimal treatment outcomes, the costs of which can range from almost nil to colossal sums when, for example, a transplanted organ is rejected[46].

The unicohort format for presenting compliance-dependent outcomes is an attractive simplification. It is not always applicable, sometimes for want of adequate data, or sometimes because (as with pharmaceuticals which have highly reliable actions—oral contraceptives, many of the antibiotics, the proton pump inhibitors) it is not a particularly useful format, simply because with such reliably acting agents the number of patients who benefit approaches the number treated.

REFERENCES

1. Urquhart J. The electronic medication event monitor—lessons for pharmacotherapy. *Clin Pharmacokinet* **32**: 345–56, 1997.
2. Harter JG, Peck CC. Chronobiology: suggestions for integrating it into drug development. *Ann NY Acad Sci* **618**: 563–71, 1991.
3. Houston MC, Hodge R. Beta-adrenergic blocker withdrawal syndromes in hypertension and other cardiovascular diseases. *Am Heart J* **116**: 515–23, 1988.
4. Psaty BM, Koepsell TD, Wagner EH, LoGerfo JP, Inui TS. The relative risk of incident coronary heart disease associated with recently stopping the use of beta blockers. *JAMA* **263**:1653–7, 1990.
5. Anon. Long-term use of beta blockers: the need for sustained compliance. *WHO Drug Information* **4**(2): 52–3, 1990.
6. Rangno RE, Langlois S. Comparison of withdrawal phenomena after propranolol, metoprolol, and pindolol. *Am Heart J* **104**: 473–8, 1982.
7. Urquhart J, Chevalley C. Impact of unrecognized dosing errors on the cost and effectiveness of pharmaceuticals. *Drug Inform J* **22**: 363–78, 1988.
8. Meyer UA, Peck CC (eds) *The Drug Holiday Pattern of Non-compliance in Clinical Trials: Challenge to Conventional Concepts of Drug Safety and Efficacy*. Washington DC: Center for Drug Development Science, Georgetown University, 1997.
9. Temple R. Dose-response and registration of new drugs. In: *Dose-Response Relationships in Clinical Pharmacology*. Eds: Lasagna L, Erill S, Naranjo CA. Amsterdam: Elsevier, 1989, pp. 145–67.
10. Potter LS. Oral contraceptive compliance and its role in the effectiveness of the method. In: *Compliance in Medical Practice and Clinical Trials*. Eds: Cramer JA, Spilker B. New York: Raven Press, 1991, pp. 195–207.
11. Guillebaud J. Any questions. *BMJ* **307**: 617, 1993.
12. Berman R. Patient compliance of women taking estrogen replacement therapy. *Drug Inform J* **31**: 71–83, 1997.
13. Anon. *Environmental campaign reveals sources and causes of unused medications*. Canada Newswire Press Release, July 16, 1996.
14. Cramer JA, Spilker B (eds) *Compliance in Medical Practice and Clinical Trials*. New York: Raven Press, 1991.
15. Steiner JF, Prochazka AV. The assessment of refill compliance using pharmacy records: methods, validity, and applications. *J Clin Epidemiol* **50**: 105–16, 1997.

16. Wasson J, Gaudette C, Whaley F, Sauvigne A, Baribeau P, Welch HG. Telephone care as a substitute for routine clinical follow-up. *JAMA* **267**: 1788–93, 1992.
17. Kass MA, Gordon M, Meltzer DW. Can ophthalmologists correctly identify patients defaulting from pilocarpine therapy? *Am J Ophthalmol* **101**: 524–30, 1986.
18. Cramer JA, Scheyer RD, Mattson RH. Compliance declines between clinic visits. *Arch Intern Med* **150**: 1509–10, 1990.
19. Feinstein AR. On white-coat effects and the electronic monitoring of compliance. *Arch Intern Med* **150**: 1377–8, 1990.
20. Petri H, Leufkens H, Naus J, Silkens R, van Hessen P, Urquhart J. Rapid method for estimating the risk of acutely controversial side effects of prescription drugs. *J Clin Epidemiol* **43**: 433–9, 1990.
21. Schneider M-P, Iorillo D, Fallab C-L, Pechère A, Chiarello N, Waeber B, Brunner H-R, Burnier M. Combined ambulatory blood pressure and electronic compliance monitoring in the management of treatment resistant hypertension. A prospective observational study. Poster, Drug Information Association Conference on Patient Non-compliance, Baltimore MD, USA, December 8, 1997.
22. Urquhart J, Heilmann K. *Risk Watch—The Odds of Life*. New York: Facts on File, 1984.
23. Urquhart J. When outpatient drug treatment fails: identifying non-compliers as a cost-containment tool. *Med Interface* **6**: 65–73, 1993.
24. Probstfield JL. Clinical trial prerandomization compliance (adherence) screen. In: *Compliance in Medical Practice and Clinical Trials*. Eds: Cramer JA, Spilker B. New York: Raven Press, 1991, pp. 323–33.
25. Urquhart J. Patient compliance as an explanatory variable in four selected cardiovascular trials. In: *Patient Compliance in Medical Practice and Clinical Trials*. Eds: Cramer JA, Spilker B. New York: Raven Press, 1991, pp. 301–22.
26. Cramer J, Vachon L, Desforges C, Sussman NM. Dose frequency and dose interval compliance with multiple antiepileptic medications during a controlled clinical trial. *Epilepsia* **36**: 1111–17, 1995.
27. Coronary Drug Project Research Group. Influence of adherence to treatment and response of cholesterol on mortality in the coronary drug project. *N Engl J Med* **303**:1038–41, 1980.
28. Horwitz RI, Viscoli CM, Berkman L, Donaldson RM, Horwitz SM, Murray CJ, Ransohoff DF, Sindelar J. Treatment adherence and risk of death after a myocardial infarction. *Lancet* **336**: 542–5, 1990.
29. Horwitz RI, Horwitz SM. Adherence to treatment and health outcomes. *Arch Intern Med* **153**: 1863–8, 1993.
30. Sackett DL, Gent M. Controversy in counting and attributing events in clinical trials. *N Engl J Med* **301**: 1410–12, 1979.
31. Lee YJ, Ellenberg JH, Hirta DG, Nelson KB. Analysis of clinical trials by treatment actually received: is it really an option. *Stat Med* **10**: 1595–1605, 1991.
32. Meier P. Discussion of dose-response estimands. *J Am Stat Assoc* **86** (413): 19–22, 1991.
33. Cox D. Discussion. *Stat Med* **17**: 387–9, 1998.
34. Efron B. Foreword. Limburg Compliance Symposium. *Stat Med* **17**: 249–50, 1998.
35. Hasford J. Biometric issues in measuring and analyzing partial compliance in clinical trials. In: *Compliance in Medical Practice and Clinical Trials*. Eds: Cramer JA, Spilker B. New York: Raven Press, 1991, pp. 265–81.
36. Feinstein AR. Intent-to-treat policy for analyzing randomized trials: statistical distortions and neglected clinical challenges. In: *Compliance in Medical Practice and Clinical Trials*. Eds: Cramer JA, Spilker B. New York: Raven Press, 1991, pp. 359–70.
37. Efron B. Rejoinder. *J Am Stat Assoc* **86** (413): 25–6, 1991.

38. Sheiner LB, Rubin DB. Intention to treat analysis and the goals of clinical trials. *Clin Pharmacol Ther* **57**: 6–15, 1995.
39. The Lipid Research Clinics Coronary Primary Prevention Trial results: (I) Reduction in incidence of coronary heart disease; (II) The relationship of reduction in incidence of coronary heart disease to cholesterol lowering. *JAMA* **251**: 351–74, 1984.
40. Manninen V, Elo MO, Frick H, Haapa K, Feinon-en OP, Heinsalmi P, Helo P, Huttunen JK, Kaitaniemi P, Koskinen P, Mäenpää H, Malkonen M, Manttari M, Norola S, Pasternack A, Pikkarainen J, Romo M, Sjoblom T, Nikkila EA. Lipid alterations and decline in the incidence of coronary heart disease in the Helsinki Heart Study. *JAMA* **260**: 641–51, 1988.
41. Levy G. A pharmacokinetic perspective on medicament non-compliance. *Clin Pharmacol Ther* **54**: 242–4, 1993.
42. Lasagna L, Hutt PB. Health care, research, and regulatory impact of non-compliance. In: *Compliance in Medical Practice and Clinical Trials.* Eds. Cramer JA, Spilker B. New York: Raven Press, 1991, pp. 393–403.
43. Urquhart J. Pharmaco-economic perspectives on patient compliance with prescribed drug regimens. *Proceedings of the European Symposium on Pharmaco-economics, Gent, 18–20 May, 1994.* European Society for Clinical Pharmacology, 1995, pp. 244–250.
44. Rich MW, Beckham V, Wittenberg C, Leven CL, Freedland KE, Carney RM. A multidisciplinary intervention to prevent the readmission of elderly patients with congestive heart failure. *N Engl J Med* **333**: 1190–5, 1995.
45. West JA, Miller NH, Parker KM, Senneca D, Ghandour G, Clark M, Greenwald G, Heller RS, Fowler MB, DeBusk RF. A comprehensive management system for heart failure improves clinical outcomes and reduces medical resource utilization. *Am J Cardiol* **79**: 58–63, 1997.
46. Aswad S, Devera-Sales A, Zapanta R, Mendez R. Costs for successful vs failed kidney transplantation: a two-year follow-up. *Transplant Proc* **25**: 3069–70, 1993.

10

Rational Prescribing in Suboptimal Compliance

Bernard Waeber, Michel Burnier, and Hans R. Brunner

Division of Hypertension and Vascular Medicine, Lausanne University Hospital, Switzerland

THE NEED FOR BETTER BLOOD PRESSURE CONTROL IN HYPERTENSIVE PATIENTS

Hypertension is a major risk factor for cardiovascular diseases[1], and lowering the blood pressure with antihypertensive drugs reduces the incidence of complications such as stroke and myocardial infarction[2]. Most patients with high blood pressure require lifelong treatment. This is not easy because hypertension is most often asymptomatic and, unfortunately, any antihypertensive medication will occasionally cause adverse reactions. Some patients may feel better when untreated than during long-term therapy.

The difficulty in treating hypertension is reflected by the fact that in less than 50% of patients prescribed antihypertensive medications is the blood pressure normalized[3,4]. This poor blood pressure control is most likely to be the main obstacle in achieving optimal protection against cardiovascular events. There is strong evidence that the blood pressure achieved by antihypertensive therapy is a better predictor of cardiovascular risk than the level before treatment[5].

POOR COMPLIANCE AS A CAUSE OF INADEQUATE BLOOD PRESSURE CONTROL

In a recent European survey, poor compliance with prescribed medications was the reason given by 70% of treating physicians for treatment failures[6]. Interestingly, the patients themselves advanced poor compliance as the determinant of inadequate blood pressure control much less frequently (16%). This mismatch between the subjective views of physicians and patients shows how difficult it is to deal with the problem of compliance in the everyday

Drug Regimen Compliance: Issues in Clinical Trials and Patient Management.
Edited by J.-M. Métry and U.A. Meyer. © 1999 John Wiley & Sons Ltd.

patient–doctor relationship. How well or how badly hypertensive patients adhere to long-term antihypertensive treatment is still largely unknown. There is, however, convincing evidence that suboptimal compliance with the prescribed regimen is associated with increased frequency of treatment failure[7]. Also, underutilization of antihypertensive drugs enhances the rate of hospitalization[8].

ASPECTS OF COMPLIANCE WITH ANTIHYPERTENSIVE THERAPY

In considering long-term pharmacological treatment of hypertension, three different steps can be identified: the adoption, the execution and the discontinuation process[9].

When drug treatment is first proposed to a patient, the initial step is a process that can be called 'adoption', in which the patient concurs with the treatment plan and agrees to undertake the proposed treatment. The patient's understanding of hypertension, the risk that it poses, and the role of the prescribed drug regimen are crucial for high rates of adoption and, for the most part, the patient's decision to adopt the proposed treatment plan occurs when the patient is together with the physician. The patient's receipt of the dispensed drug from the pharmacist and administration of the first dose can be regarded as the end of the adoption process and the point of transition to the second. During this phase poor communication, low motivation from the doctor or the patient (or both), and socioeconomic barriers might influence adversely the outcome of long-term compliance[10].

The second process, referred to as the 'execution' process, corresponds to the day-to-day taking of the prescribed dose at the prescribed time(s). The execution process belongs to the patient's daily life, away from the physician and other caregivers. Efforts should be directed during this stage to help the patient by various compliance enhancement strategies[11]. For example, a key point is to find for each individual patient a treatment that is at the same time efficacious and well tolerated. Hypertensive patients perceiving problems during their treatment tend to modify the prescribed drug regimen spontaneously, either by lowering the dosage or by taking fewer medications than instructed[12].

Finally, there should be few, and only medical, reasons for discontinuing treatment that is meant to be lifelong. In reality a substantial proportion of patients treated for hypertension decide, for various reasons, to discontinue treatment. A few years ago, it was estimated that 50% of patients with hypertension drop out of care within a year[13]. This figure may be too pessimistic, but it is crucial to reinforce the patient's motivation during long-term treatment. In this respect it is essential to learn as much as possible about the patient's habits in medication taking, as a declining compliance might be a signal of impending discontinuation.

THE 'EXECUTION' PROCESS OF COMPLIANCE

During the 'execution' process compliance can be regarded as the extent to which the patient's actual dosing history corresponds to the prescribed regimen. Compliance as such is therefore not just the percentage of prescribed doses taken but also involves consideration of the intervals between doses, and the extent to which some intervals may be longer than the drug's duration of action, in which case drug action is interrupted.

It is now possible to monitor compliance using electronic medication dispensers that record each time the container is opened. Most of the experience accumulated so far with 'real-time' compliance has been obtained using electronic medication event monitoring[14]. However, the antihypertensive drug trials that have used this device have been of rather short duration (a few weeks to a few months)[15-18].

The most frequent error is a delay in dosing—e.g. the usually taken morning dose is postponed until evening. The next most commonly seen error is to skip a single dose which, in once-daily dosing regimens, means an interval between doses of 48 hours or more. The third most common error is to skip two sequential doses, which, in once-daily dosing regimens, means an interval between doses of 72 hours or more. Then come longer lapses in dosing, called drug holidays, in which dosing is interrupted for three or more days. Drug holidays occur less often than the shorter lapses, but (of course) entail longer periods without drug action, interrupting the action of even the longest-acting of the presently used drugs. Thus, the usual claim of '24–hour control' for once-daily antihypertensive drugs does not tell how well the product can be expected to control blood pressure when these most common errors occur.

How important is the duration of drug activity considering the fact that the day-to-day compliance with treatment is often not perfect? A prospective crossover study was performed in a general practice environment to assess and compare compliance data obtained by electronic monitoring, for two calcium antagonists, one given twice a day (slow-release nifedipine) and the other one once a day (amlodipine), in 113 patients with hypertension or stable angina pectoris[18]. Each treatment period lasted 4 weeks. Table 10.1 shows the number of patients taking the drug as prescribed.

TABLE 10.1 Number of patients correctly taking the prescribed drug for at least 90%, 80–90% or 80% of the observed days[18]

One dose/day	Two doses/day			Total
	≥90%	80–90%	≤80%	
≥90%	50	12	17	79
80–90%	6	6	12	24
≤80%	1	0	9	10
Total	57	18	38	113

The proportions of the treatment periods with insufficient drug activity at several hypothetical levels of duration of drug effect, based on the actual timing of drug intake observed during the two phases of the study, was then calculated. Figure 10.1 illustrates, for each hour of a 24–h period, the percentage of days with insufficient drug activity when the hypothetical duration of

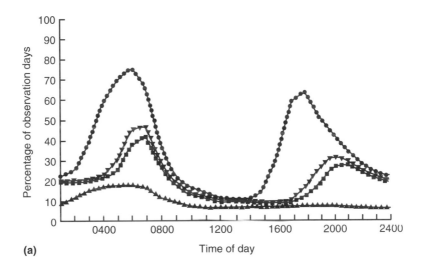

(a)

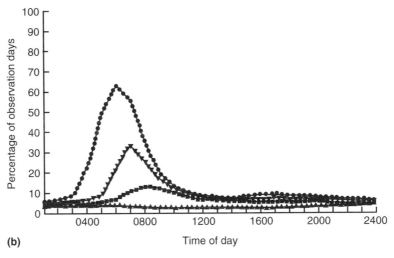

(b)

Figure 10.1 Percentage of days with insufficient drug activity during the 24-h period according to various hypothetical durations of action, based on actual timings of drug intake in all patients. (a) Twice-daily administration (hypothetical drug action: ●–● 9 h; ▼–▼ 11.5 h; ■–■ 12 h; ▲–▲ 18 h); (b) drug administration once a day (hypothetical drug action: ●–● 21 h; ▼–▼ 23 h; ■–■ 24 h; ▲–▲ 36 h). From ref 18, with permission.

drug action was 9, 11.5, 12 or 18 h for a twice-daily regimen, and 21, 23, 24 and 36 h for a once-daily regimen. The uncovered period tended to peak in the early morning for a single daily dose with a duration of action of 24 h or less, and relatively minor decreases in this duration (from 24 to 21 h) were accompanied by a relatively large increase in this peak. For the twice-daily regimen, and for all tested durations of action (except for 18 h), two peaks of uncovered time were apparent, the morning peak being more pronounced than the evening peak.

TYPICAL COMPLIANCE PATTERNS

The profile of a perfect complier is shown in Figure 10.2(a). The patient was asked to take one blood pressure-lowering tablet each day. He actually did so

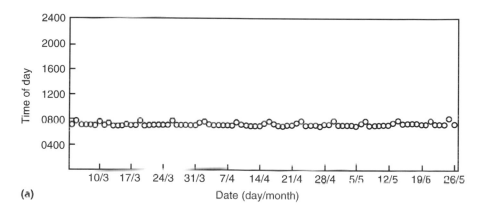

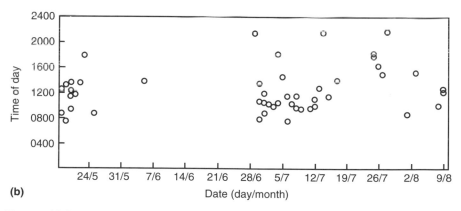

FIGURE 10.2 Examples of compliance patterns. (a) A perfect complier; (b) a poor complier

for the 3-month monitoring period, and opened the box at almost the same time every day.

The patient profiled in Figure 10.2(b) was also prescribed a once-daily medication for 3 months. He showed, however, a very erratic pattern. Only 26% of doses were taken, with large variations in timing. The patient also omitted doses for periods from several days to several weeks. Of note is that the patient occasionally took 1–3 extra doses per day.

These two examples have been gathered from a trial carried out by practising physicians[19]. The patients were informed about the proper use of the electronic device and knew that their compliance with the prescribed drug would be monitored. It is therefore impressive to see how the compliance behavior can differ from patient to patient, even during a short-term follow-up.

PERSPECTIVE ON MONITORING COMPLIANCE

Compliance with antihypertensive treatment is a key determinant of blood pressure control and thereby of the prevention of cardiovascular morbidity and mortality. It is difficult for a physician to ascertain whether a patient is a good or a poor complier. Thus, the physician's estimated compliance rate is only weakly correlated with the compliance rates obtained by objective measure or by electronic monitoring[20]. Most non-compliers go undetected by their physician and are most often misjudged as 'non-responders'. If properly identified, such patients could be encouraged to improve their compliance. The objective record of the patient's dosing history appears to be a valuable tool for detecting the kinds of errors a patient is making and to document progress towards the goal of satisfactory compliance. This approach should not be regarded as an intrusion in the privacy of the patient's life, but as a privileged occasion of discussion between patient and physician. Of note, the objective record makes the patient accountable for achieving improvements.

CONCLUSIONS

The electronically compiled dosing record appears to be a useful tool for assessing patients' actual dosing stories, to pinpoint the nature of dosing errors, and to guide efforts to achieve and maintain adequate compliance, which is expected to improve the long-term quality of blood pressure control.

REFERENCES

1. MacMahon, S., R. Peto, J. Cutler, R. Collins, P. Sorlie, J. Neaton, R. Abbot, J. Godwin, A. Dyer, and J. Stamler. 1990. Blood pressure, stroke, and coronary heart disease. Part I. Prolonged differences in blood pressure: prospective observational studies corrected for the regression, dilution bias. *Lancet* **335**:765–777.
2. Collins, R., R. Peto, S. MacMahon, P. Hebert, N. H. Fiebach, K. A. Eberlein, J. Godwin, N. Qizilbash, J. O. Taylor, and C. H. Hennekens. 1990. Blood pressure, stroke and coronary heart disease. Part 2. Short-term reductions in blood pressure: overview of randomized drug trials in their epidemiological context. *Lancet* **335**:827–838.
3. Burt, V. L., J. A. Cutler, M. Higgins, M. Horan, D. Labarthe, P. K. Whelton, C. Brown, and E. J. Rocella. 1995. Trends in prevalence, awareness, treatment and control of hypertension in the adult US population: data from the health examination surveys 1960–1991. *Hypertension* **26**:60–69.
4. Mancia, G., R. Sega, C. Milesi, G. Cesana, and A. Zanchetti. 1997. Blood-pressure control in the hypertensive population. *Lancet* **349**:454–457
5. Isles, C. G., L. M. Walker, and G. D. Beevers. 1986. Mortality in patients of the Glasgow Blood Pressure Clinic. *J. Hypertens.* **4**:141–156.
6. Ménard, J. and G. Chatellier. 1995. Limiting factors in the control of blood pressure: why is there a gap between theory and practice. *J. Hum. Hypertens.* **9** (suppl 2):19–23.
7. Rudd, P. 1995. Clinicians and patients with hypertension: unsettled issues about compliance. *Am. Heart J.* **130**:572–579.
8. Maronde, R. F., L. S. Chan, F. J. Larssen, L. R. Strandberg, M. F. Laventurier, and S. R. Sullivan. 1989. Underutilization of antihypertensive drugs and associated hospitalization. *Med. Care* **27**:1159–1166.
9. Waeber, B., H. R. Brunner, and J. M. Métry. 1997. Compliance with antihypertensive treatment: implications for practice. *Blood Pressure* **6**:326–331.
10. Breckenridge, A. 1983. Compliance of hypertensive patients with pharmacological treatment. *Hypertension* **5** (suppl III):85–89.
11. Miller, N. H., M. Hill, T. Kottke, and I. S. Ockene. 1997. The multilevel compliance challenge: recommendations for a call to action. A statement for healthcare professionals. *Circulation* **95**:1085–1090.
12. Wallenius, S. H., K. K. Vainio, M. J. H. Korhonen, A. G. Hartzema, and H. K. Enlund. 1995. Self-initiated modification of hypertension treatment in response to perceived problems. *Ann. Pharmacother.* **29**:1213–1217
13. Eraker, F. A., J. P. Kirscht, and M. H. Becker. 1984. Understanding and improving patient compliance. *Ann. Intern. Med.* **100**:258.
14. Urquhart, J. 1997. The electronic medication event monitor—lessons for pharmacotherapy. *Clin. Pharmacokinet* **32**:345–356.
15. Rudd, P., S. Ahmed, V. Zachary, C. Barton, and D. Bonduelle. 1990. Improved compliance measures: applications in an ambulatory hypertensive drug trial. *Clin. Pharmacol. Ther.* **48**:676–685.
16. Mallion, J. M., B. Meilhac, F. Tremel, R. Calvez, and N. Bertholom. 1992. Use of a microprocessor-equipped tablet box in monitoring compliance with antihypertensive treatment. *J. Cardiovasc. Pharmacol.* **19** (suppl. 2):42–48.
17. Kruse, W., J. Rampmaier, G. Ullrich, and E. Weber. 1994. Patterns of drug compliance with medications to be taken once and twice daily assessed by continuous electronic monitoring in primary care. *Int. J. Clin. Pharmacol. Res.* **32**:452–457.
18. Waeber, B., P. Erne, H. Saxenhofer, and G. Heynen. 1994. Role of drugs with duration of action greater than 24 hours. *J. Hypertens.* **12** (suppl 8):67–71.

19. Waeber, B., Vetter, W., Darioli, R., Keller, U., Brunner, H.R. Improved blood pressure control by monitoring compliance with antihypertensive therapy (submitted for publication).
20. Rudd, P., Y. Ramesh, C. Bryant-Kosling, and D. Guerrero. 1993. Gaps in cardiovascular medication taking: the tip of the iceberg. *J. Gen. Intern. Med.* **8**:659–666.

11

The Role of Compliance in Clinical Care

Dieter Magometschnigg

Gesellschaft für Klinische Pharmakologie, Kinderspitalgasse, Wien, Switzerland

INTRODUCTION

Clinical trials are in many basic aspects different from routine patient care. It is therefore inadmissible to assume that interventions performed in routine patient care will come up with exactly the results that were found in clinical trials addressing a similar clinical question. Clinical trials are carefully planned and strictly designed experiments to give an answer to a very distinct clinical question: whether a certain dose of a certain drug is more potent than placebo. In order to get an unbiased answer, all the conditions that might alter the parameter to be studied must be defined. Therefore inclusion and exclusion criteria are used to select a highly homogenous sample of participating subjects. The subjects are stratified and allocated randomly to experimental and control groups. Most importantly, the method used to study a certain effect must be qualified. It is essential that the method used varies only within an acceptable range and gives highly reproducible results. The electronic medication event monitoring system is the most reliable method of measuring compliance[1-4].

Routine patient care is not intended to yield scientific results. It is, or should be, the practical application of the insights acquired by clinical trials. Consequently the patients and the methods and goals of patient management are often very different from those of clinical trials. Nothing is defined, designed, stratified or allocated randomly and even the diagnostic procedures differ. As a rule, clinical routine work differs essentially from the respective clinical studies to such an extent that it is always uncertain whether a study result can be transferred into clinical care, or whether findings in patient care can be proven in clinical trials.

COMPLIANCE IN CLINICAL TRIALS

Ever since medical professionals began to advise patients their advice has been ignored, partly or wholly—even Hippocrates complained about non-

Drug Regimen Compliance: Issues in Clinical Trials and Patient Management.
Edited by J.-M. Métry and U.A. Meyer. © 1999 John Wiley & Sons Ltd.

compliance. Nowadays the best method to ensure that a patient takes a prescribed drug is still an unsolved problem. Even under the best conditions guaranteed in clinical studies compliance is incomplete. If we compare profiles of the compliance measured by electronic monitoring (the most reliable method currently available), we see a rather uniform behaviour of patients[3,5,6]: only about 80% of the stratified and randomized participants comply satisfactorily (i.e. given instructions are followed by 80%). Even under optimal conditions 20% of the study population don't follow the protocol. If this behaviour is not recognized, at least 20% of untreated patients will be considered as treated and therefore bias the study results.

Compliance data are needed in order to avoid erroneous conclusions of trial results. High levels of non-compliance in a clinical trial increase the risk of a type 2 error. For a comparative study with a power of 95% to show a difference between two groups at the 5% level and to accommodate a mean compliance of 50%, the number of subjects in each group must be increased about fourfold[7-9].

Clinical trials are rarely set up to study compliance itself. As a rule, efficacy is the primary goal and compliance is often measured additionally, just to reduce the bias of missing effects caused by lacking drug intake. If a study is designed to answer the question 'do hypertensive patients treated by a T1-receptor antagonist cough rarely, compared to a control group taking an ACE-inhibitor?' the outcome of this study, concerning compliance, cannot be extrapolated to the hypertensive population as a whole, even if MEMS was used.

In summary, the overall compliance of participants in clinical trials is about 80%. Transferring these results to patients treated in a routine setting would lead to an untrue conception of the reality.

COMPLIANCE IN CLINICAL CARE

Investigating compliance in clinical routine work is much more difficult than measuring drug intake during a clinical trial, especially if the extent of compliance is the primary goal of the study. In order to prevent observer bias, each investigation of drug intake must keep the conditions of clinical care constant. The random sample of patients studied must not be selected by any criteria and the patients' behaviour must not be altered by the survey itself.

It is unclear whether informing a patient about the goal of a compliance study (to study his behaviour of drug intake and of dispensing the questionable drug in an electronically monitored package instead of the industrial standard packaging) will influence the patient's behaviour or not. The observer bias becomes worse if, in order to obtain additional information about the consequences of non-compliance, one also tries to take into consideration an efficacy parameter. The higher the differences between investigational procedure and care are in order to avoid biased efficacy results, the less information about care we can expect. Consequently, when investigating compliance the biasing conditions of routine care cannot be modified, and efficacy results must be biased.

In order to give an example of the problems addressed in studying compliance in routine patient care, two studies will be discussed in this chapter.

Trial 1

In order to investigate compliance of drug intake in hypertensives, treated by general practitioners in their daily routine, cilazapril was dispensed in an electronically monitored package. To avoid observer bias, no restrictions were made by any kind of specific protocol and blood pressure was measured as usual by participating physicians. The investigation was performed in 1803 patients, who were treated by 389 general practitioners[10].

The analysis of compliance and blood pressure demonstrated two important facts:

1. More than half of the patients were poor or non-compliers; only 40% of the patients took more than 75% of the prescribed drug.
2. The fall in blood pressure, which was measured by casual readings as usual, was the same in compliant (systolic/diastolic pressure 25/16 mmHg) and in non-compliant (systolic/diastolic: 27/18 mmHg) patients.

Thus we must conclude that:

1. Compliance of patients treated by general practitioners is poor, much lower than compliance of study participants (approximately 80%).
2. The assessment of blood pressure by casual readings, as it is done in routine work, is insufficient to measure treatment effects as fall in blood pressure was the same in compliers and non-compliers.
3. Consecutively judging routinely taken blood pressures as a means for targeting possible non-compliers via their failing drug response is an insufficient tool.

Trial 2

A second trial was designed to study if self-recording of blood pressure enhanced compliance. All the participating patients were treated with enalapril[11]. After 2 months of treatment the patients were fully informed about the aim of the investigation. They were allocated to two groups, one that would self-record blood pressure and one that would not. The enalapril was dispensed in an electronically monitored package to both groups. A total of 147 hypertensive patients, who took their blood pressure twice a day for at least one month with the blood-pressure monitor provided (and after having undergone training in blood pressure self-recording), was compared with 175 patients who did not monitor their own blood pressure. Both groups were treated by their general practitioners.

The analysis of the study data gave completely different results from the results of Trial 1.

1. Compliance exceeded 80% and was the same in both groups. We believe this high level was caused by investigator bias. Informing the patients about the aims of this investigation extensively promoted drug intake.
2. Blood pressures as measured by the general practitioners were the same in both groups. There was no additional decrease during the period of the survey. However, even if compliance had been increased by the influence of the observers, this effect would not have been detected by routinely performed casual readings, as the first study had shown.
3. Self-recorded blood pressures, in contrast, did fall in the survey period (systolic/diastolic: by 10/8 mmHg).

SUMMARY

A combination of addressing the topic of compliance to the patient and close follow-up enhances compliance in patients treated by the general practitioner to a level similar to that known for study participants. Routine control of blood pressure is an insufficient tool for detecting treatment effects. Obviously a method showing a fall in blood pressure in up to 40% of patients treated with placebo in clinical trials is an insufficient guide for identifying non-compliant patients.

Who is the Hypertensive in whom Compliance should be Measured?

As the common way of blood pressure recordings is inappropriate to find out if a treatment is effective, it cannot be helpful in deciding in whom compliance should be measured. Preselection of patients who should be given priority for supervision has not been possible because we have no clinical hint to distinguish between compliers and non-compliers. Compliance in chronic treatment is known to fall within the first 3 months, and data on compliance after 3–6 months of treatment should be offered to patients who desire objective control of drug intake.

To exclude at least some patients from compliance measuring, for reasons of cost and practical efficiency, we must turn the question around and ask 'in which patients is measurement of compliance senseless?' In patients who do not want to cooperate or patients who feel that measuring of compliance is exposing them to a 'police watchdog', measurement of compliance could cause loss of confidence in treatment. Whether responders to treatment could be excluded from studies is questionable; patients apparently responding to treatment cannot be identified as non-compliers.

Economic Implications

The economic consequences of non-compliance in non-responders are obvious[4,12]: drugs are prescribed and paid for, but the condition of the patient does not improve. Consequently additional diagnostic procedures are performed, additional therapies are prescribed and hypertension will cause end-organ damage. Therefore we can conclude that, as qualified treatment is a request of healthcare, solving of the non-compliance problem is crucially important. In hypertensives in whom non-compliance was only 50%–86%[12], the cost of termination or interruption of newly initiated episodes of anti-hypertensive drug therapy were compared with those of continuous drug intake by a regression analysis comparing total healthcare cost minus cost of prescription drugs[13,14]. Continuous therapy was estimated to save approximately US$3 per patient per day. The magnitude of the estimated saving led to the Omnibus Budget Reconciliation Act of 1990, which encouraged the development of methods to measure real-time drug profiles of a patient's drug therapy[15].

Costs are also incurred by non-compliant patients who are misjudged as effectively treated. These patients do not take the prescribed drugs but are not at risk of end-organ damage. However, as long as a physician is unaware that the improvement is not due to the treatment, he or she will continue to observe the patient, to prescribe drugs, to control treatment risks—and thus increase costs.

Institutions Suited to Measure Compliance

Compliance monitoring depends on special equipment, which must be operated by trained staff. The drugs must be supplied in special drug containers, which can only be done by a pharmacist. Patients must be informed about the importance, the meaning and the advantages of compliance. Analysis of the drug containers and communication with the patient and the physician is again the task of a specially trained staff. Only some institutions could meet these requirements.

1. The pharmacist who dispenses the drug is the best person to supervise patient compliance. The patient might feel better if the prescriber and the institution controlling their behaviour are not the same, especially as non-compliance has a negative touch.
2. A physician carrying out compliance supervision may face a dilemma. On one hand the physician is responsible for prescribing and controlling chronic drug treatment, and therefore needs to know whether the patient is taking a prescribed drug in the recommended way. On the other hand the patient should be free to give, or not to give, information about drug compliance to the doctor. Responsibility on the one hand, and free decision of the patient on the other, may conflict when the physician is controlling compliance.
3. Independent institutions specialising in patient services could also fulfil the task of controlling compliance without conflicting the freedom of the patient's decision to inform, or not to inform, the physician of drug intake.

Steps Necessary for Implementing Compliance Control in Clinical Routine

Cheaper and more sophisticated compliance measuring devices are needed, especially instruments suitable for controlling a multiple drug regimen. All the involved healthcare partners should be appropriately aware of the importance of non-compliance.

The patient should learn to accept compliance measurement as a valuable treatment service and the physician should learn to use compliance control as an aid to control treatment. Health services should take into account that supporting this system is cheaper than uncontrolled drug prescription, and the pharmaceutical industry must accept that their investment in advertisements is lost in non-compliant patients. As cost-effectiveness of drug treatment depends on drug intake, improving compliance enhances efficacy of treatment and optimizes the investment of all the healthcare partners.

How to Approach Non-compliance?

A patient recognized as non-compliant should be given assistance to improve this unwelcome behaviour. Today several techniques are offered[16], but only a few have been used in clinical trials and possibly none has been questioned for its efficacy in a controlled compliance study.

In the trial discussed earlier in this chapter on whether compliance in hypertensives can be improved by blood pressure self-recording[10], an investigator bias was caused by informing both the contributing physicians and the patients about the aim of the study and its procedures. These precautions were followed by compliance of 80%, a rate similar to that seen in most clinical trials. The study did not answer the addressed question as both study groups had a high rate of full compliance. Despite this we can take into account that addressing and thoroughly controlling compliance is a simple technique.

The question of which strategies might simply and effectively improve non-compliance cannot yet be answered. Controlled trials are needed to learn how we can proceed.

Outlook

Compliance control should be integrated into clinical routine; the technical equipment necessary has already been implemented. We need a lobby interested in promoting this topic and powerful enough to be heard by the health services, pharmacists, general physicians and patients.

REFERENCES

1. Rudd P, Ahmed S, Zachary V *et al.* Improved compliance measures: application in an ambulatory hypertensive drug trial. *Clin Pharmacol Ther* 1990; **48:** 676–685.
2. Pullar T, Kumar S, Tindall H, Feely M. Time to stop counting the tablets. *Clin Pharmacol Ther* 1989; **46:** 163–168.
3. Cramer JA, Mattson RH, Prevey ML, Scheyer RD, Quellett VL. How often is medication taken as prescribed? A novel assessment technique. *JAMA* 1989; **261:** 3273–3277.
4. Urquhart J, Chevalley C. Impact of unrecognised dosing errors on the cost effectiveness of pharmaceuticals. *Drug Inform J* 1988; **22:** 363–378.
5. De Clerk E, van der Linden S. Compliance monitoring of NSAID drug therapy in ankylosing spondylitis: experiences with an electronic monitoring device. *Br J Rheumatol* 1996; **35:** 60–65.
6. Kass MA, Melter D, Gordon M *et al.* Compliance with topical pilocarpine treatment. *Am J Ophthalmol* 1986; **101:** 515–523.
7. Feinstein AR. Clinical biostatistics. Biostatistical problems in 'compliance bias'. *Clin Pharmacol Ther* 1974; **16:** 846–857.
8. Feinstein AR. 'Compliance bias' and the interpretation of clinical trials. In: Hynes RB, Tayler DW, Sackett DL eds. *Compliance in health care.* Baltimore: John Hopkins University Press, 1979; 360–377.
9. Goldsmith CH. The effect of differing compliance distribution on the planning and statistical analysis of therapeutical trials. In: Sackett DL, Haynes RB eds. *Compliance with therapeutic regimens.* Baltimore: Johns Hopkins University Press, 1976; 137–151.
10. Magometschnigg D, Neumann K. Compliance of hypertensive patients treated by their family doctors. *Int J Clin Pharmacol Ther* 1994; **32:** 152.

11. Magometschnigg D, Hitzenberger G. Die Compliance des Hypertonikers in der ärztlichen Praxis-Analys einer Anwendungsbeobachtung 2. Teil 1997; **22:** 525–528.

12. Hasford J. Compliance and the benefit/risk relationship of antihypertensive treatment. *J Cardiovasc Pharmacol* 1992; **20:** 30–34.

13. Col N, Fanale EJ, Kronholm P. The role of medication noncompliance and adverse drug reactions in hospitalization of elderly. *Arch Intern Med* 1990; **150:** 841–845.

14. McCombs JS, Nichol MD, Newman CM, Sclar DA. The costs of interrupting antihypertensive drug therapy in a Medicaid population. *Med Care* 1994; **32:** 214–226.

15. US Government. *Omnibus Budget Reconciliation Act of 1990.* Washington DC: US Government Printing Office, 1990.

16. Spilker B. Methods of assessing and improving patients compliance in clinical trials. In: Cramer AJ, Spilker B, eds. *Patient compliance in medical practice and clinical trials.* New York: Raven Press, 1991; 37–56.

17. SHEP Cooperative Research Group. Prevention of stroke by antihypertensive drug treatment in older persons with isolated systolic hypertension: final results of the Systolic Hypertension in the Elderly Program (SHEP). *JAMA* 1991; **256:** 3255–64.

12

Behavioral Strategies for Long-term Survival of Transplant Recipients

Sabina De Geest[1,2], Ivo Abraham[2,3], Jacqueline Dunbar-Jacob[4], and Johan Vanhaecke[1]

[1]Leuven Heart Transplant Program, University Hospitals KU-Leuven, Belgium; [2]Center for Health Services and Nursing Research, School of Public Health, Catholic University of Leuven, Belgium; [3]The Epsilon Group, Charlottesville, VA, USA; [4]Center for Research in Chronic Disorders, School of Nursing, University of Pittsburgh, PA, USA

INTRODUCTION

The successes in transplantation over the last two decades (e.g. advances in immunosuppression, surgical techniques and other aspects of patient management) have increased survival and quality of life after solid organ transplantation. However, long-term success remains compromised by the side-effects of the immunosuppressive drugs, chronic rejection, and graft loss due to late acute rejection episodes. It is being recognized that lifelong follow-up is as much a psychosocial and behavioral as it is a physiological health process. The psychological and behavioral dimensions are evident from the mere fact that post-transplant life requires a number of lifelong compliance behaviors: medication-taking, infection prevention, self-monitoring for signs of infection and rejection, avoidance of risk factors for cardiovascular disease, following guidelines for alcohol use, regular clinic visits, and yearly check-up examinations. Failure to comply with this therapeutic regimen may result in increased morbidity and mortality, and in excessive healthcare expenditures. In particular, not taking immunosuppressive medication as prescribed can be devastating because lifelong immunosuppression is a prerequisite for good graft function. Non-compliance with immunosuppressive therapy may cause late acute rejection, graft loss, and even death.

This chapter will discuss the importance of non-compliance with immunosuppressive regimen as a limiting factor in long-term success after solid organ transplantation. The development of preventive and restorative

Drug Regimen Compliance: Issues in Clinical Trials and Patient Management.
Edited by J.-M. Métry and U.A. Meyer. © 1999 John Wiley & Sons Ltd.

interventions to reduce the risk for non-compliance with immunosuppressive therapy should build upon determinants of non-compliance in transplant populations. Relevant patient-related, treatment-related factors and variables related to the provider and healthcare setting with regard to non-compliance will be summarized. Three sets of behavioral strategies for enhancing long-term survival after solid organ transplantation will be discussed—strategies to initiate the therapeutic regimen, strategies to maintain medication adherence, and strategies to remedy compliance problems.

CLINICAL SIGNIFICANCE OF NON-COMPLIANCE WITH IMMUNOSUPPRESSION

The negative impact of non-compliance on clinical outcome has been documented by case reports in renal, heart, and liver transplant recipients since the early days of transplantation. Analysis of larger cohorts of transplant patients also revealed that non-compliance with immunosuppressive medication is a major cause of late acute rejection episodes and graft failure in solid organ transplant recipients[1–16].

Two approaches can be identified in assessing non-compliance with immunosuppressive therapy in transplant populations. A first approach refers to *subclinical non-compliance*. This is the assessment of non-compliance with immunosuppressive therapy in the absence of major clinical complications at time of compliance measurement. This approach contrasts with the study of *clinical non-compliance*, in which non-compliance is assessed in relation to the occurrence of a clinical event such as a rejection episode, graft loss, or death. Clinical non-compliance is only the proverbial tip of the iceberg and captures only a small proportion of the actual non-compliers. In contrast, subclinical non-compliance focuses on the iceberg as a whole, as it enables us to detect all non-compliant patients, regardless of their present clinical status. Assessing subclinical non-compliance is most valuable in unraveling the effects of a transplant patient's non-compliance with the immunosuppressive therapy on clinical outcome[2,3,5].

Two research projects focusing on subclinical non-compliance conducted at the University Hospitals of Leuven have documented the unequivocal relationship between transplant patients' non-compliance with immunosuppressive drugs and negative outcome more than one year after transplantation. A first descriptive cross-sectional study[2] investigated the prevalence, determinants, and consequences of subclinical non-compliance with immunosuppressive therapy in 148 adult Caucasian renal transplant recipients with more than one year post-transplant status. Of these, 84 were men and 64 were women, with a mean age of 46 years (range 18–69). Time since transplantation ranged from 12 to 228 months[2]. Non-compliance with immunosuppressive therapy was assessed using self-reports and patients were categorized as non-compliers when they admitted during interviews to have skipped immunosuppressive medication on a regular basis over the last 12 months (i.e. having missed several doses a month or taking 'drug holidays').

The renal transplant study revealed that the prevalence of subclinical non-compliance with immunosuppressive therapy was 22.3%. Late acute rejection incidence, defined as rejection episodes more than one year post-transplant, was only 6% in the compliant group but 24% in the non-compliant group ($p = 0.003$). Actuarial graft survival at 5 years was 98.7% for the compliers and 93.6% for the non-compliers, a significant difference ($p = 0.03$). No significant difference was found in terms of the occurrence of chronic rejection episodes or in terms of patient survival at 5 years[2].

The results of the renal transplant study stimulated us to proceed in our efforts to unravel the relationship between transplant patients' compliance behavior and clinical outcome. More specifically, the next step was to determine the clinical risk associated with varying *degrees* of subclinical non-compliance. We therefore refined our methodology by using a more sophisticated longitudinal design to better study the dynamics of change over time. In addition, we opted for a more reliable and sensitive measurement method of assessing non-compliance with the immunosuppressive regimen. Self-report (as used in the renal transplant study), pill count, assay, and collateral report all have major methodological drawbacks[3,17]. A technologically more advanced and sophisticated method of assessing non-compliance with immunosuppressive medication is electronic event monitoring[3,17,18]. This method uses a pill bottle fitted with a cap with a microelectronic circuit that registers bottle opening and closing. Stored event data are downloaded to a computer, which is used to generate listings and graphics, allowing the detection of patterns and visualization of the dynamics of medication behavior. Electronic event monitoring holds promise as a potential 'gold standard' for medication compliance measurement. It shows more sensitivity than other methods[18,19], and it allows continuous level and multidimensional compliance measurement. Still, electronic event monitoring remains an indirect method because ingestion remains unproved[9,17,18].

Using electronic event monitoring, we longitudinally assessed subclinical non-compliance with cyclosporine (CsA) therapy during a 3-month period in 101 Caucasian adult heart transplant recipients (14 women, 87 men). Patients had a median age of 56 (range 51–61) years, and a median post-transplant status of 3 (range 1 6) years[3,5]. Using iterative partitioning methods of cluster analysis, including non-standardized electronic event monitoring compliance parameters, patients were categorized by degree of subclinical cyclosporine-non-compliance into a three-cluster solution. Overall compliance was high, with a median of 99.4%. The three derived clusters (excellent compliers (84%), minor subclinical non-compliers (7%) and moderate subclinical non-compliers (9%)) differed significantly by degree of subclinical non-compliance ($p<0.0001$) and showed a 1.19%, 14.28%, and 22.22% incidence of late acute rejections ($p = 0.01$), respectively. These results showed that, although in absolute numbers CsA-compliance in this sample was high, minor deviations from dosing schedule (>3%), too large variations in dosing intervals, and/or the occurrence of drug holidays (no medication intake for more than 24 hours) were associated with an increased risk for acute late rejection episodes. These findings underscore the pivotal role of patients' compliance in successful long-term outcome after transplantation and suggest the minimal tolerance for deviation from a prescribed medication regimen of CsA[3,5].

We also assessed *clinical non-compliance* in our heart transplant study. More specifically, we determined whether non-compliance with immunosuppressive therapy was an etiological factor in the occurrence of the ten late acute rejection episodes (>1 year post-transplant) in our series using both electronic event monitoring and self-report data[3,4,20]. Non-compliance appeared to be an influential causative factor in nine of the ten acute late rejection episodes occurring in five non-compliers, indicating that non-compliance with immunosuppressive therapy is a major risk factor in the etiology of acute late rejections after cardiac transplantation.

The significance of non-compliance with immunosuppressive therapy as a major behavioral risk factor for negative outcome more than 1 year after heart transplantation is further suggested by a recent analysis of the International Society of Heart and Lung Transplantation Registry data. It appears that 9% of the mortality more than 1 year after transplant in this registry is due to acute late rejection episodes[21]. Although this analysis does not elucidate the etiology of these rejection episodes, it is likely that the contribution of non-compliance is considerable.

This evidence shows manifestly that non-compliance with the immunosuppressive regimen constitutes a particular challenge for healthcare workers in dealing with transplant populations. Reliable and valid assessment of non-compliance based on a sound operational definition and measurement method is a prerequisite for studying determinants of non-compliance with immunosuppressive therapy among transplant recipients. Knowledge of determinants is critical for developing preventive interventions to diminish the risk for non-compliance as well as restorative interventions to enhance compliance in transplant populations.

It is of utmost importance to develop patient profiles to identify patients at risk, to develop and implement preventive interventions to diminish the risk for non-compliance and to develop restorative interventions to enhance compliance in transplant populations in order to improve long-term survival after solid organ transplantation. Development of compliance interventions should build upon the available evidence regarding determinants of non-compliance in the transplant compliance literature.

DETERMINANTS OF NON-COMPLIANCE IN TRANSPLANT RECIPIENTS

Determinants of non-compliance can be categorized into patient-related factors, treatment-related factors, and variables related to the provider and the healthcare setting.

Patient-related Factors

Demographic characteristics such as gender, race, and social class have shown limited value in predicting non-compliance in transplant populations. The transplant literature reveals that patients over the age of 40 are at a lower risk for non-compliance behavior than adolescent transplant recipients, who show the highest rate of non-compliance[6,8,9,22–29].

A major determinant of future compliance with drug treatment is *past compliance* and *compliance at initiation of the medication regimen*[30]. Pretransplant or previous non-compliance appeared to be a reliable clinical predictor for post-transplant non-compliance in heart[5,15,31] and renal[6,8,28,32,33] transplant recipients. Evidence from the transplant literature indicates that appointment non-compliance and medication non-compliance are related in some fashion[3,5,6,8,28,33–36]. Appointment non-compliance is easy to detect and should therefore be regarded as a warning signal for medication non-compliance in clinical practice.

Lack of adequate knowledge has to be regarded as an important cause of non-compliance[37]. Patients need to understand the nature of their regimen and the purpose of their medications. They need to know what kind of behaviors the therapeutic regimen requires, how and when to perform them, and what to do if problems arise. For instance, situational–operational knowledge, defined as problem-solving abilities and strategies, is negatively associated with non-compliance in renal transplant recipients[2]. Soine *et al.*[38] have reported a negative correlation between heart transplant recipients' knowledge levels and the number of reported rehospitalizations. Although transplant recipients may show improvement in neurocognitive functioning after transplantation[39], severe *cognitive impairment* in the early post-transplant course due to hepatic encephalopathy, steroid psychosis, infectious diseases, or cerebral hypoperfusion may compromise the patient's ability to benefit from education and to independently manage his or her medication regimen[39–42].

There is reasonably strong research evidence linking *social support* and patient compliance[43]. Studies on compliance behavior in transplant[12,23,34,44–47] and non-transplant[48–52] populations have suggested the beneficial effect of social support (e.g. significant others preparing the patient's medication for administration, reminding patients to take their medication punctually, redeeming prescriptions, and assisting in deciding to contact a healthcare worker when problems arise) on health-related behaviors and outcomes. Received (rather than perceived) informational, tangible, emotional and appraisal support facilitates compliance with medication regimens[43,53]. The relationship between the patient and healthcare worker may also be a source of social support. There are indications that patient satisfaction in general and satisfaction with regard to the relationship between the healthcare worker and the patient in particular, positively influence compliance[54].

Social isolation is a risk factor for non-compliance, not only because of a lack of social support but because of a higher prevalence of depressive symptomatology in socially isolated individuals[55]. Depressive symptoms negatively influence illness representations[56] and consequent coping behavior in relation to compliance with therapeutic regimens[57]. The sense of inadequacy in performing activities of daily life common in depressed patients contributes to non-compliance with therapeutic regimen.

Marital status, more specifically not being in a stable relationship with a partner, is a rough measure of social isolation and has been identified as a risk factor for non-compliance in transplant recipients[2–4,20,33,44,46]. Empirical evidence suggests that both pretransplant and post-transplant psychiatric morbidity negatively influences compliance with medical regimen[15,31,36,58,59]. More specifically, studies indicate a significant relation between preoperative[6,36,60] and current[12,28,45,46,61–63] psychiatric status and postoperative compliance in transplant recipients.

It is important to emphasize the relevance of patients' common sense as a potential trigger for non-compliance with therapeutic regimens (cf. Common Sense Model[64]). Common sense refers to dynamic cognitive structures that can be adjusted by new experiences, by information from the mass media, and through communications with healthcare workers[64]. Patient perceptions about their illness and treatment, and their symptom experience, affect their compliance and health behavior; for instance, non-compliance with antihypertensive medications because the patient is convinced that he or she 'can feel when my blood pressure is up' and takes their medicine only when they notice that they have 'high blood pressure'. Incongruity between a patient's common sense and a healthcare worker's therapeutic recommendations is a major cause of intentional non-compliance.

Immunosuppressive drugs carry side-effects that have been identified as a possible cause of non-compliance[6,28,29], yet it is rather the patient's subjective appraisal of symptom distress associated with adverse events or side-effects that triggers non-compliance[64–66]. Cosmetic side-effects of immunosuppressive drugs, although they have limited relevance in terms of morbidity and mortality, may be highly distressing in female transplant recipients and may trigger non-compliance. Subjective symptom experience is rarely part of clinical examinations and is infrequently evaluated in clinical trials. However, subjective symptom distress is an invaluable clinical parameter in quality of life assessments and in determining patients at risk for non-compliance[67].

Self-efficacy is an important determinant in non-compliance research, not only because efficacy beliefs are predictive of future health behavior[68], but also because self-efficacy is influenced by clinical intervention. Self-efficacy expectations are defined as the perception that one can master certain tasks or perform adequately in given situations[69]. Self-efficacy was found to be a determinant of non-compliance with immunosuppressive therapy in both our renal and heart transplant studies[2,5]. Self-efficacy beliefs are generated from four sources. *Performance accomplishments* are the most influential source of self-efficacy information and are based on authentic mastery experiences. *Vicarious experience* refers to learning that occurs through observation of events and/or other people (e.g. role modeling). *Verbal persuasion* and related types of social influences denote processes to strengthen people's beliefs that they possess certain capabilities and is frequently used in patient education programs. *Physiological state,* being the magnitude of visceral arousal in taxing or stressful situations, is the final source of self-efficacy beliefs (e.g. anxiety inhibits learning). Self-efficacy beliefs are generated from these four sources through cognitive processing. Thus a mastery experience, being the most powerful source of efficacy perceptions, can be influential only if patients perceive success as being the result of their own effort[69–71].

Treatment-related Factors

Duration and complexity of the therapeutic regimen have been identified as major obstacles in compliance with long-term intake of medication[18,19,37,72]. Transplant recipients are prone to non-compliance because their therapeutic regimen is complex and because it has to be followed throughout life. Studies reveal that the incidence of non-compliance increases with the length of time since transplantation[29,45,46,73,74]. Compliance interventions should therefore not be limited to the immediate post-transplant period. The number of prescribed medications, a measure of complexity of a medication regimen, has been found to be positively related with non-compliance rates in renal transplant recipients[19], but other studies have not confirmed this relationship[2,3,8].

In addition to complexity and duration, cost of the medication is increasingly being identified as a determinant of non-compliance. Cost containment is a major issue in both American and European healthcare systems. The proportion of cost-sharing in the form of copayments for medications therefore increases steadily, resulting in a growing number of patients not being able to purchase the prescribed medication[75–77].

Factors Related to Provider and Healthcare Environment

Characteristics of provider and healthcare environment are the third set of determinants of non-compliance that establish the foundation for compliance interventions in transplant populations. More specifically, the healthcare worker's communication style affects patient compliance: an open and empathic approach is preferable to a dominant and judgmental style that does not take the patient's perspective into consideration. Moreover, excellent didactic skills are imperative to maximize the effect of educational interventions[78,79].

Procedural aspects of the healthcare setting are also influential on patients' compliance behavior. For instance, long waiting times in outpatient clinics, lack of continuity of care (both with regard to healthcare provider and concerning the regularity of follow-up appointments) and difficult access to healthcare all negatively influence compliance[78].

STRATEGIES TO ENHANCE LONG-TERM SURVIVAL AFTER ORGAN TRANSPLANTATION

Transplant patients deserve special attention in view of compliance with immunosuppressive therapy because compliance is critical to long-term survival after transplantation. Moreover, transplant patients show a minimal tolerance for deviation from a prescribed medication regimen of cyclosporine (see above), necessitating 100% compliance[3,5]. Nurses can play a prominent role in identifying patients at risk for non-compliance and in developing interventions to enhance compliance. However, compliance management implies multidisciplinary collaboration.

The foundations for a compliance intervention program consist of the available evidence regarding determinants of non-compliance behavior (see above) and the results of experimental studies assessing the effect of compliance interventions in transplant and non-transplant populations. Yet randomized controlled trials are scarce and methodological weaknesses such as the unreliable measurement of compliance, the lack of assessment of clinical outcome, and the limited time of follow-up for long-term treatments, preclude firm conclusions[79,80]. Compliance interventions can be categorized in three groups: (1) strategies to initiate compliance; (2) interventions to maintain compliance; and (3) interventions to remedy compliance problems[78].

Strategies to Initiate Compliance

The rationale for implementing strategies to initiate compliance in the clinical setting is based on the evidence that compliance at initiation of the medication regimen is predictive of future compliance[30]. Inadequate knowledge, skills and understanding all negatively influence compliance with drug treatment[30]. *Assessment of capacity to adhere* with medication regimen is critical. Functional and sensory abilities, cognitive functioning, literacy, knowledge, motivation, 'common sense', sources of social support and financial status must be carefully assessed at the initiation of treatment. Different strategies can be combined: (1) educational interventions; (2) behavioral interventions; (3) social support interventions.

Educational Strategies

Patient education is a crucial element in compliance management. Nurses as well as other members of the therapeutic team should educate transplant patients and their families at initiation of a therapeutic regimen regarding (1) intended effect of medication, (2) administration of medication (e.g. dose, time of administration, precautions), (3) side-effects/symptom distress of medication, and (4) monitoring of medication. Consideration should also be given as to how to implement the medication regimen in daily life and what to do in case problems arise.

A phased approach is preferable in patient education. Both oral and written information should be provided (e.g. patient education booklets, medication cards) and special materials should be developed to instruct patients with low literacy (e.g. picture schedule[81]). The use of interactive computer programs shows promise as a cost-effective tool in patient education. Formal evaluation of patient education is imperative[82].

Behavioral Strategies

Knowledge alone does not guarantee compliance. A self-medication program aiming to increase self-efficacy with medication intake, in addition to patient education strategies, increases the effectiveness of the intervention[83,84]. The purpose of a self-medication program is to increase a transplant patient's confidence in managing their medication regimen during hospitalization. The program includes strategies focused on mastery experiences (e.g. bedside management of medication regimen), role modeling (e.g. a videotape in which a transplant patient explains the importance of strict compliance and suggests strategies for compliance), and verbal persuasion (e.g. formal patient education by a healthcare worker). Finally, high levels of symptom distress, anxiety or other sources of physiological arousal may impede the acquisition of self-efficacy perceptions and should be taken into account in the development of intervention programs to enhance compliance.

Tailoring the medication regimen to the patient's lifestyle and reducing the complexity of the therapeutic regimen will enhance compliance. Self-monitoring strategies (e.g. using a medication check-off list), the use of medication aids (e.g. medication box, writing the number of daily doses on medication container lids), and cueing (e.g. leaving containers in a particular location, taking medications in association with meals or bedtime, setting alarm clocks to administer medications) are also helpful in adhering to drug treatment[78,79,85,86].

Social Support Interventions

An active involvement of the partner/family member in patient education and a self-medication program is important as social support positively influences health, well-being and compliance[55]. The interventions at initiation of treatment allow development of a therapeutic alliance between transplant patient and their family and healthcare worker. Good communication and patient satisfaction enhance compliance. Significant others must be involved in educational and behavioral interventions during the in-hospital phase. They have to be knowledgeable about the transplant patient's therapeutic regimen and must be informed on how they can facilitate compliance (see above). Partners can function as a role model after a patient's discharge from hospital (cf. self-efficacy and social support) and thus support the patient in his or her compliance efforts.

Critical Pathways/Case Management

The initiation of a drug regimen is complex and is the responsibility of the whole multidisciplinary transplant team. Evaluation is mandatory throughout the transplant process. The use of critical pathways[87] and case management[88] are helpful to streamline compliance management during hospitalization and after discharge in the home setting. Critical pathways refer to a clinical instrument, developed for a specific patient population, that maps care needs, structures, organizes and plans interventions, and indicates what patient outcome should be achieved in what time. Critical pathways are based on standard problems and interventions for a 'case type'. It is a network technique permitting coordination and gearing of the activities of different disciplines to one other to achieve the desired outcome. Case management 'provides outcome-oriented patient care within an appropriate length of stay, uses appropriate resources based on specific case types, promotes the integration and coordination of clinical services, monitors the use of patient care resources, supports collaborative practice and continuity of care, and enhances patient and provider satisfaction'[88].

This multidimensional approach combining educational, behavioral, and social support interventions should improve long-term compliance in daily life. Yet it is the combination of strategies that will guarantee success[78–80,86]. For instance, an experimental study using a family-based program to promote medication compliance in pediatric renal transplant recipients combined educational (verbal and written information for patients and parents), social support (peer modeling, parents involvement in the program), and behavioral strategies (role modeling (cf. self-efficacy), monitoring of medication intake (medication calendar), cueing, reminders)[89]. However, the results were inconclusive concerning the effect of the intervention on knowledge and compliance levels[89], probably due to the small sample size ($n = 29$), the unreliable compliance measurement (pill count and assay), and the lack of a comprehensive evidence-based multidimensional compliance intervention.

Maintaining Treatment Compliance

The scientific evidence from randomized controlled trials with regard to maintaining compliance is also limited[79,80,86]. Nevertheless, there is little doubt that continuity of care enhances compliance. Regular follow-up by the same healthcare worker using an open and empathic approach facilitates compliance, certainly in chronic patient populations such as transplant recipients[78–80,86]. Follow-up can be established by clinic appointments. Follow-up by telephone or the use of other communication methods (e.g. videophone, e-mail, and fax) is increasing, primarily because of their convenience and cost-effectiveness. However, their effectiveness in terms of compliance management for specific patient populations such as transplant patients should be addressed further.

Compliance must be monitored as an important clinical parameter throughout the post-transplant course. The most cost-effective strategy for routine compliance assessment is self-report, as it has been shown to effectively identify a proportion of actual non-compliers[2,3,5]. A non-threatening, non-accusatory, open-ended, and information-intensive approach is more likely to elicit a truthful answer pattern[2]. The use of more sophisticated methods such as electronic event monitoring may be indicated in some high-risk patients. Logs for self-monitoring can also be helpful for compliance screening and intervention.

Risk factors for non-compliance should also be examined carefully during transplant follow-up (e.g. appointment non-compliance, adolescence, knowledge deficit, depression, symptom distress, social isolation). Questioning the patient's perceptions concerning their illness and treatment ('common sense') may reveal obstacles to compliance[63]. Finally, the organization of follow-up care should provide easy accessibility (home healthcare) and restricted waiting time in order to enhance patient satisfaction[78,79,86].

Remedying Compliance Problems

If non-compliance with drug treatment is observed, the reason for the non-compliance should first be determined (e.g. cognitive impairment, knowledge deficit, incongruity in 'common sense', depressive symptomatology, symptom distress). This will provide a basis from which to choose the most adequate compliance interventions (counseling, patient education, self-efficacy interventions, social support strategies, etc.). Interventions should target both the transplant patient and their significant other(s). Active involvement of both the patient and the family is critical to determining those strategies and practical aids that are perceived to be most helpful to accomplish correct medication intake in daily life[79,80,86]. The use of electronic event monitoring can also be useful: it not only allows continuous compliance assessment but also permits detailed feedback to patients concerning past compliance; for instance by discussing printouts with the patient/family (cf. self-efficacy). Further studies evaluating the efficacy of electronic event monitoring and other high-tech interventions such as videophone contact in remediating adherence problems are indicated.

RESEARCH AGENDA

Future research is necessary to strengthen the scientific base for the development of compliance intervention programs. Therefore replication research concerning prevalence, determinants and consequences of non-compliance with immunosuppressive therapy for the different organ transplant populations is indicated. Although non-compliance is prevalent in all solid organ transplant populations, one wonders if the prevalence, determinants and consequences of non-compliance with immunosuppressive therapy are similar among heart, liver, and kidney transplant recipients. The use of electronic event monitoring is mandatory in compliance studies in transplant populations in order to guarantee validity and reliability of results.

A next step will be the development of patient profiles to identify patients at risk for medication non-compliance in the various organ transplant populations. Longitudinal studies starting before transplantation and following patients throughout the post-transplant course are indicated to achieve this goal. Attention should also be given to specific risk groups such as pediatric transplant recipients.

Testing the effectiveness of compliance interventions in randomized clinical trials will provide the strongest evidence for clinical practice. Intervention studies should also include a cost analysis in order to determine both the cost of non-compliance and the cost of interventions. Multicenter studies might provide an understanding of transplant center effects on compliance as well as the influence of healthcare systems (e.g. accessibility, cost reimbursement) on behavioral outcome after transplantation.

Transplant nursing has a pivotal role in the further improvement of the long-term survival of transplant recipients. Focusing on the behavioral aspects of the transplant process is a prerequisite in doing so.

REFERENCES

1. Addonizio LJ, Hsu DT, Smith CR, Gersony WM, Rose EA. Late complications in pediatric cardiac transplant recipients. *Circulation* 1990; **82** (suppl IV): IV295–IV301.
2. De Geest S, Borgermans L, Gemoets H, Abraham I, Vlaminck H, Evers G, Vanrenterghem Y. Incidence, determinants, and consequences of subclinical noncompliance with immunosuppressive therapy in renal transplant recipients. *Transplantation* 1995; **59**: 340–347.
3. De Geest S. *Subclinical non-compliance with immunosuppressive therapy in heart transplant recipients. A cluster analytic study*. Doctoral dissertation, School of Public Health, Catholic University of Leuven, Belgium, 1996.
4. De Geest S, Abraham I, Vanhaecke J. Comparison of patient characteristics of clinical noncompliers and clinical compliers with immunosuppressive therapy after heart transplantation. *European Heart Journal, Abstract Supplement* 1996; **17**: 37.
5. De Geest S, Abraham I, Moons P, Vandeputte M, Van Cleemput J, Evers G, Daenen W, Vanhaecke J. Late acute rejections and subclinical non-compliance with cyclosporine-therapy in heart transplant patients. *Journal of Heart and Lung Transplantation* 1998; **17**: 854–863.
6. Didlake RH, Dreyfus K, Kerman RH, Van Buren CT, Kahan BD. Patient noncompliance: a major cause of late graft failure in cyclosporine-treated renal transplants. *Transplantation Proceedings* 1988; **10** (Suppl. 3): 63–69.
7. Douglas JF, Hsu DT, Addonizio LJ. Non-compliance in pediatric heart transplant patients. *Journal of Heart and Lung Transplantation* 1993; **12**: S92.
8. Dunn J, Golden D, Van Buren CT, Lewis RM, Lawen J, Kahan BD. Causes of graft loss beyond two years in the cyclosporine era. *Transplantation* 1990; **49**: 349–353.
9. Ettenger RB, Rosenthal JT, Marik JL, Malekzadeh M, Forsythe SB, Kamil ES, Salusky IB, Fine RN. Improved cadaveric renal transplant outcome in children. *Pediatric Nephrology* 1991; **5**: 137–142.
10. Hilbrands LB, Hoitsma AJ, Koe RAP. Medication compliance after renal transplantation. *Transplantation* 1995; **60**: 914–920.
11. Hong JH, Sumrani N, Delaney V, Davis R, Dibenedetto A, Butt KMH. Causes of late renal allograft failure in the Ciclosporin era. *Nephron* 1992; **62**: 272–279.
12. Kiley DJ, Lam CS, Pollak R. A study of treatment compliance following kidney transplantation. *Transplantation* 1993; **55**: 51–56.
13. Malekzadeh M, Pennisi A, Uittenbogaart C, Korsch BM, Fine RN, Main ME. Current issues in pediatric renal transplantation. *Pediatric Clinics of North America* 1976; **23**: 857–872.
14. Mor E, Gonwa TA, Husberg BS, Goldstein RM, Klintmalm GB. Late-onset acute rejection in orthotopic liver transplantation—associated risk factors and outcome. *Transplantation* 1992; **54**: 821–824.
15. Paris W, Muchmore J, Pribil A, Zuhdi N, Cooper DKC. Study of the relative incidence of psychosocial factors before and after heart transplantation and the influence of post-transplantation psychosocial factors on heart transplantation outcome. *Journal of Heart and Lung Transplantation* 1994; **13**: 424–432.
16. Troppmann C, Benedetti E, Gruessner RWC, Payne WD, Sutherland DER, Najarian JS, Matas AJ. Retransplantation after renal allograft loss due to noncompliance. Indications, outcome, and ethical concerns. *Transplantation* 1995; **59**: 467–471.
17. De Geest S, Abraham I, Dunbar-Jacob J. Measuring transplant patients' compliance with immunosuppressive therapy. *Western Journal of Nursing Research* 1996; **18**: 595–605.

18. Cramer JA, Mattson RH, Prevey ML, Scheyer RD, Ouellette VL. How often is medication taken as prescribed? A novel assessment technique. *JAMA* 1989; **261**: 3273–3277.
19. Cheung R, Dickins J, Nicholson PW, Thomas ASC, Smith HH, Larson HE, Deshmukh AA, Dobbs RJ, Dobbs SM. Compliance with anti-tuberculous therapy: a field trial of a pill-box with a concealed electronic recording device. *European Journal of Clinical Pharmacology* 1988; **35**: 401–407.
20. De Geest S, Abraham I, Dunbar-Jacob J, Vanhaecke J. The significance of noncompliance in the etiology of acute late rejections in the heart transplant population. *Circulation* 1997; **96** (Abstract Supplement): I-15.
21. Hosenpud JD, Bennett LE, Keck BM, Fiol B, Novick RJ. The Registry of the International Society for Heart and Lung Transplantation: Fourteenth official report. *Journal of Heart and Lung Transplantation* 1997; **16**: 691–712.
22. Armstrong SH, Weiner MF. Non-compliance with post-transplant immunosuppression. *International Journal of Psychiatry in Medicine* 1981; **11**: 89–95.
23. Beck DE, Fennell RS, Yost RL, Robinson JD, Geary D, Richards GA. Evaluation of an educational program on compliance with medication regimens in pediatric patients with renal transplants. *Journal of Pediatrics* 1980; **96**: 1094–1097.
24. Fine RN, Malekzadeh MH, Pennisi AJ, Ettenger RB, Uittenbogaart CH, Vida F, Negrete RN, Korsch BM. Long-term results of renal transplantation in children. *Pediatrics* 1978; **61**: 641–650.
25. Foulkes LM, Boggs SR, Fennell RS, Skibinski K. Social support, family variables, and compliance in renal transplant children. *Pediatric Nephrology* 1993; **7**: 185–188.
26. Gagnadoux MF, Niaudet P, Broyer M. Non-immunological risk factors in paediatric renal transplantation. *Pediatric Nephrology* 1993; **7**: 89–95.
27. Hesse UJ, Roth B, Knuppertz G, Wienand P, v. Lilien T. Control of patient compliance in outpatient steroid treatment of nephrologic disease and renal transplant recipients. *Transplantation Proceedings* 1990; **22**: 1405–1406.
28. Schweitzer RT, Rovelli M, Palmeri D, Vossler E, Hull D, Bartus S. Non-compliance in organ transplant recipients. *Transplantation* 1990; **49**: 374–377.
29. Sketris I, Grobler M, West M, Gerus S. Factors affecting compliance with cyclosporine in adult renal transplant recipients. *Transplantation Proceedings* 1994; **26**: 2538–2541.
30. Dunbar J. Predictors of patient adherence. Patient characteristics. In: Shumaker SA, Schron EB, Ockene JK (Eds). *The handbook of health behavior change*. Springer, New York, 1990, pp. 348–360.
31. Levenson JL, Olbrisch ME. Psychosocial evaluation of organ transplant candidates. A comparative survey of process, criteria, and outcomes in heart, liver, and kidney transplantation. *Psychosomatics* 1993; **34**: 314–323.
32. Ramos EL, Kasiske BL, Alexander SR, Danovitch GM, Harmon WE, Kahana L, Kiresuk TJ, Neylan JF. The evaluation of candidates for renal transplantation. *Transplantation* 1994; **57**: 490–497.
33. De Geest S, Abraham I, Vanhaecke J. Clinical risk associated with appointment non-compliance in heart transplant recipients. *Circulation* 1996, **94** (Abstract Supplement): I-180.
34. Rodríguez A, Diaz M, Cólon A, Santiago-Delpin EA. Psychosocial profile of noncompliant transplant patients. *Transplantation Proceedings* 1991; **23**: 1807–1809.
35. Meyers KEC, Weiland H, Thomson PD. Paediatric renal transplantation noncompliance. *Pediatric Nephrology* 1995; **9**: 189–192.
36. Shapiro PA, Williams DL, Foray AT, Gelman IS, Wukich N, Sciacca R. Psychosocial evaluation and prediction of compliance problems and morbidity after heart transplantation. *Transplantation* 1995; **60**:1462–1466.

37. Meichenbaum D, Turk DC. Factors affecting adherence. In: Meichenbaum D, Turk DC (Eds). *Facilitating treatment adherence. A practitioner's guide book.* Plenum Press, New York–London, 1987, pp. 41–70.
38. Soine L, Cunningham S, Shaver J, Gallucci B. Knowledge level of rejection, immunosuppressive therapy, infection and myocardial biopsy of heart transplant recipients and their significant support persons. *Journal of Heart and Lung Transplantation* 1992; **11**: 196.
39. Riether AM, Smith S, Lewison BJ, Cotsonis GA, Epstein CM. Quality-of-life changes and psychiatric and neurocognitive outcome after heart and liver transplantation. *Transplantation* 1992; **54**: 444–450.
40. Balthazor JE. Steroid psychoses and hepatic encephalopathy in liver transplant patients: which is which and what do you do? *Critical Care Nursing Quarterly* 1991; **14**: 51–55.
41. Freeman AM, Folks DG, Sokol RS, Fahs JJ. Cardiac transplantation: clinical correlates of psychiatric outcome. *Psychosomatics* 1988; **29**: 47–54.
42. Surman OS. Psychiatric aspects of liver transplantation. *Psychosomatics* 1994; **35**: 297–307.
43. Levy RL. Social support and compliance: update. *Journal of Hypertension* 1985; **3**: 45–49.
44. Cooper DKC, Lanza RP, Barnhard CN. Non-compliance in heart transplant recipients: the Cape Town experience. *Journal of Heart Transplantation* 1984; **3**: 248–253.
45. Dew MA, Roth LH, Thompson ME, Kormos RL, Griffith BP. Medical compliance and its predictors in the first year after heart transplantation. *Journal of Heart and Lung Transplantation* 1996; **15**: 631–645.
46. Frazier PA, Davis-Ali SH, Dahl KE. Correlates of non-compliance among renal transplant recipients. *Clinical Transplantation* 1994; **8**: 550–557.
47. Korsch BM, Fine RN, Negrete VF. Non-compliance in children with renal transplants. *Pediatrics* 1978; **61**: 872–876.
48. Christensen AJ, Smith TW, Turner CW, Holman JM, Gregory MC, Rich MA. Family support, physical impairment, and adherence in hemodialysis: an investigation of main and buffering effects. *Journal of Behavioral Medicine* 1992; **15**: 313–325.
49 Doherty NJ, Schrott HG, Metcalf L, Laslello Vailas L. Effect of spouse support and health beliefs on medication adherence. *Journal of Family Practice* 1983; **17**: 837–841.
50. Hubbard P, Muhlenkamp AF, Brown N. The relationship between social support and self-care practices. *Nursing Research* 1984; **33**: 266–270.
51. Mermelstein R, Cohen S, Lichtenstein E, Baer JS, Kamarck T. Social support and smoking cessation and maintenance. *Journal of Consulting and Clinical Psychology* 1986; **54**: 447–453.
52. Muhlenkamp AF, Sayles JA. Self-esteem, social support, and positive healthcare practices. *Nursing Research* 1986; **35**: 334–338.
53. Aaronson LS. Perceived and received support: effects on health behavior during pregnancy. *Nursing Research* 1989; **38**: 4–9.
54. DiMatteo MR, DiNicolla DD. *Achieving patient compliance: the psychology of the medical practitioner's role.* Pergamon Press, New York, 1982.
55. Turner RJ, Marino F. Social support and social structure: a descriptive epidemiology. *Journal of Health and Social Behavior* 1994; **35**: 193–212.
56. Salovey P, Birnbaum D. Influence of mood on health relevant cognitions. *Journal of Personality and Social Psychology* 1989; **57**: 539–551.
57. Franks P, Campbell TL, Shields CG. Social relationships and health: the relative roles of family functioning and social support. *Social Science and Medicine* 1992; **34**: 779–788.

58. Frierson RL, Lippman SB. Heart transplant candidates rejected on psychosocial grounds. *Psychosomatics* 1987; **28**: 347–355.
59. Phipps L. Psychiatric aspects of heart transplantation. *Canadian Journal of Psychiatry* 1991; **36**: 536–568.
60. Mai FM, McKenzie FN, Kostuk WJ. Psychosocial adjustment and quality of life following heart transplantation. *Canadian Journal of Psychiatry* 1990; **35**: 223–227.
61. Ruygrok PN, Agnew TM, Coverdale HA, Whitfield C, Lambie NK. Survival after heart transplantation without regular immunosuppression. *Journal of Heart and Lung Transplantation* 1994; **13**: 208–211.
62. Santiago-Delpín E, González Z, Morales-Otero L, Cruz N, Rive-Mora E, Amadeo JH, Acosta-Otero A, Perez JO. Transplantation in Hispanics: the Puerto Rico experience. *Transplantation Proceedings* 1989; **21**: 3958–3960.
63. Ueling DT, Hussey JL, Weinstein AB, Wank R, Bach FH. Cessation of immunosuppression after renal transplantation. *Surgery* 1976; **79**: 278–281.
64. Leventhal H, Diefenbach M, Leventhal EA. Illness cognition: using common sense to understand treatment adherence and affect cognition interactions. *Cognitive Therapy and Research* 1992; **16**: 143–163.
65. Moons P, De Geest S, Abraham I, Van Cleemput J, Vanhaecke J. Symptom experience associated with maintenance immunosuppression after heart transplantation: patients' appraisal of side-effects. *Heart and Lung* 1988; **27**: 315–325.
66. Moons P, De Geest S, Mekers G, Vanhaecke J. Symptoomervaring bij hart-transplantatiepatiënten: Een verpleegkundig aandachtsgebied. *Cordiaal* 1997; **3**: 77–79.
67. Anderson RB, Testa MA. Symptom distress checklist as a component of quality of life measurement: comparing prompted reports by patient and physician with concurrent adverse events report via the physician. *Drug Informational Journal* 1994; **28**: 89–114.
68. O'Leary A. Self-efficacy and health. *Behavioral Research Therapy* 1985; **23**: 437–451.
69. Bandura A. Human agency in social cognitive theory. *American Psychologist* 1989; **44**: 1175–1183.
70. Bandura A. *Social foundations of thought and action*. Prentice Hall, Englewood Cliffs, NJ, 1986.
71. Schneider MS, Friend R, Whitaker P, Wadhwa NK. Fluid non-compliance and symptomatology in end-stage renal disease: cognitive and emotional variables. *Health Psychology* 1991; **10**: 209–215.
72. Haynes RB. Determinants of compliance: the disease and the mechanics of treatment. In: Haynes RB, Taylor DW, Sackett DL (Eds). *Compliance in healthcare*. Johns Hopkins University Press, Baltimore, 1979, pp. 49–62.
73. Beresford TP, Schwartz J, Wilson D, Merion R, Lucey MR. The short-term psychological health of alcoholic and non-alcoholic liver transplant recipients. *Alcoholism: Clinical and Experimental Research* 1992; **16**: 996–1000.
74. Grady KL, Russell KM, Srinivasan, Constanzo MR, Pifarre R. Patient compliance with annual diagnostic testing after heart transplantation. *Transplantation Proceedings* 1993; **25**: 2978–2980.
75. Roth HP. Problems with adherence in the elderly. In: Shumaker SA, Schron EB, Ockene JK (Eds). *The handbook of health behavior change*. Springer, New York, 1990, pp. 315–326.
76. Sisson S, Tripp J, Paris W, Cooper DKC, Zuhdi N. Medication compliance and its relationship to financial factors after heart transplantation. *Journal of Heart and Lung Transplantation* 1994; **13**: 930.
77. Slymen DJ, Drew JA, Williams SJ. Determinants of non-compliance and attrition in the elderly. *International Journal of Epidemiology* 1996; **25**: 411–419.

78. Burke LE, Dunbar-Jacob J. Adherence to medication, diet, and activity recommendations: from assessment to maintenance. *Journal of Cardiovascular Nursing* 1995; **9**: 62–79.
79. Dunbar–Jacob J, Burke LE, Puczynski S. Clinical assessment of adherence to medical regimens. In: Nicassio PM, Smith TW (Eds). *Managing chronic illness: A biopsychosocial perspective*. American Psychiatric Association, Washington DC, 1995, pp. 313–349.
80. Haynes RB, McKibbon KA, Kanani R. Systematic review of randomized trials of interventions to assist patients to follow prescriptions for medications. *Lancet* 1996; **348**: 383–386.
81. Hussey LC. Minimizing effects of low literacy on medication knowledge and compliance among the elderly. *Clinical Nursing Research* 1994; **3**: 132–144.
82. Houston-Miller N, Taylor CB. *Lifestyle management for patients with coronary heart disease*. Current Issues in Cardiac Rehabilitation Series, Monograph Number 2. Human Kinetics, Champaign, 1995, pp. 21–30.
83. Lowe CJ, Raynor DK, Courtney EA, Purvis J, Teale C. Effects of self-medication programme on knowledge of drugs and compliance with treatment in elderly patients. *British Medical Journal* 1995; **310**: 1229–1231.
84. Traiger CL, Bui LL. A self-medication program for transplant recipients. *Critical Care Nurse* 1997; **17**: 71–79.
85. Conn V, Taylor S, Miller R. Cognitive impairment and medication adherence. *Journal of Gerontological Nursing* 1994: 41–47.
86. Rogers PG, Bullmann R. Prescription medicine compliance: a review of baseline of knowledge—A report of the National Council on Patient Information and Education. In: Fincham J. (Ed.). *Advancing prescription medicine compliance. New paradigms, new practices*. Haworth Press, Binghampton NY, 1995, pp. 3–36.
87. Epping P, Goossens W, Jacobs T. Het kritische pad, een geïntegreerde manier van zorgplanning. *Tijdschrift voor verpleegkundigen* 1996; **11**: 329–332.
88. Cohen E, Cesta T. Overview of health care trends. In: *Nursing case management: From concept to evaluation*. Mosby, St. Louis, 1993, pp. 3–10.
89. Fennell RS, Foulkes LM, Boggs SR. Family based program to promote medication compliance in renal transplant children. *Transplantation Proceedings* 1994; **26**: 102–103.

13

Commercial Implications of Reliable Patient Information

Guy Heynen

Pfizer AG, Zurich, Switzerland

Correct usage is a fundamental prerequisite for the realization of full value from any product. The less complex consumer products typically have relatively simple instructions for use, plus a substantial margin for errors in usage. Indeed, a basic design criterion for most consumer products is simplicity and obviousness of proper usage, plus a wide tolerance for deviations from ideal usage. One sees these characteristics in, for example, computer operating systems designed for the mass market, where the earlier strict requirements for one precise command to execute each step have been replaced by a multiplicity of different ways to accomplish a particular maneuver, all facilitated by vivid graphics, a network of help messages, and suggested next steps. Another example is provided by automobiles designed for general use, which are able to maintain predictable, stable handling in the face of substantially suboptimal steering and braking by inexpert drivers. Of course, the cars designed for aficionados are designed for optimal performance and are correspondingly much less forgiving of inexpert driving, to the point of being dangerous in the hands of the 'Sunday driver'.

It is easy to regard prescription pharmaceuticals as very special products that have little or no correspondence with other types of consumer products and are, as such, exempt from the basics that constrain all consumer products. The sense of uniqueness hinges on several key points: the drug is prescribed by a specially educated and licensed professional with whom the consumer has a special, private relationship, and the consumer is not a neutral, independently acting individual, but a patient who is ill and in need of medical help—quite different from the man who goes into a shop to buy a garden hose. These special factors have contributed to the long-standing sense that the pharmaceutical industry has unique status.

Yet many social changes in the past several decades have altered many aspects of the doctor–patient relationship, and with it the nature of

Drug Regimen Compliance: Issues in Clinical Trials and Patient Management.
Edited by J.-M. Métry and U.A. Meyer. © 1999 John Wiley & Sons Ltd.

prescription drugs. In the USA, for example, the *Physicians' Desk Reference* is a best-selling book, which patients purchase so they can learn all the 'secrets' that in past times were accessible only to caregivers. The World Wide Web has exploded with a profusion of medical information that is freely available to whoever cares to access it. Patient groups abound, oriented around particular diseases and agitating for change, including faster access to new drugs. The increasingly liberal conversion of prescription drugs to over-the-counter availability is one of many signs that these are indeed consumer products. In many countries with long-standing reputations for stringent, risk-averse drug regulation, for example, some of the biggest-selling prescription pharmaceuticals (e.g. ibuprofen, cimetidine, ranitidine) are now sold over the counter.

Another set of forces for altered perspectives comes from some very basic changes in the pharmaceutical marketplace. In the early 1960s, the requirement for proof of efficacy in properly controlled trials was imposed as a precondition for registration in the technically advanced countries. At that time, the pharmaceutical market could be characterized as having relatively few products of proven effectiveness, sold at relatively low prices. Today, many sectors of the pharmaceutical market have many products of proven effectiveness, sold at relatively high prices. The claim that a pharmaceutical is new, proven effective, and without blemish on its safety record (so far), no longer has the automatic appeal that it once had, because the market has grown in sophistication and is now looking for what one can best call 'proof of value'.

Concepts of pharmaceutical value are discussed in Chapter 9, but suffice it to say here that the mere fact of pharmacoeconomics having become a topic of consideration in respect to each newly registered pharmaceutical product is a very basic change in the market. The discussion of the various ways in which poor and partial compliance can influence pharmacoeconomic assessment is, of course, another dimension that must now be reckoned with.

Even with all these changes, the assertion that a prescription pharmaceutical is a 'consumer product' may ruffle some professional feathers. Be that as it may, we have long since passed the point where physicians could automatically assume that their instructions were routinely lucid and fully understood by patients, and that all patients (perhaps with the exception of a cantankerous or mentally deranged few) would naturally follow those instructions to the letter. The physician–patient relationship has evolved from an authoritarian 'doctor knows best' to what some like to call a 'therapeutic partnership', in which the doctor has the burden of convincing a skeptical patient to accept a proposed treatment plan, usually accompanied by a welter of questions from the patient. Such questions in an earlier time would often have been viewed as, if not rude, at least out of place, for the proper response was expected to be warm thanks and payment for the visit. The visit ended with the physician giving the patient the prescription(s), and trusting that the patient would indeed 'do as doctor says'.

Now we find ourselves with extensive, objective records of how patients actually take, or do not take, their prescribed medications in ambulatory care.

It is yet another step away from the old authoritarian mode, and it has, not surprisingly, caught some physicians unawares—clearly evident when one happens to be with the doctor when he or she first sees dosing histories of patients long assumed to be fully compliant. It brings, one might say, yet another form of realism into the doctor–patient relationship.

From the pharmaceutical marketing perspective we are now confronted, as never before, by the full extent to which our products are misused by patients in the course of ambulatory care. It is not a message everyone wants to receive. This new information has impact all the way up the line from the beginnings of human trials of a new ambulatory-care drug, through registration, and into the market.

The question of how we present evidence for the therapeutic action of a drug has gained a new perspective from the realization that common lapses in dosing in a large minority of patients can result, in those patients, in relatively small degrees of dose-dependent drug actions, simply because the doses they take are lower than prescribed. Meanwhile, the essentially correctly dosing majority get the full dose-dependent action. Then, when we average the responses across all patients, as the intention-to-treat (ITT) policy would have us do, we get an intermediate value of drug efficacy that is not characteristic of the recommended dose, and that is characteristic of a few patients whose drug intake happens to be toward the upper end of the spectrum of partial compliance. That tells us something, but it seems hardly the 'flagpole of certainty amidst the chaos', as Efron describes ITT analysis[1]. A more pragmatic approach would be to take a leaf from the American labeling of cholestyramine[2], and give the effectiveness and safety data from all patients, from good compliers, and from two or three subgroups who make the most common errors in compliance. Among other things, such labeling would reveal the relative sensitivity of each product to the more common lapses in dosing—i.e. missing a single dose, or two days of consecutively missed doses.

EXPERIENCES WITH ELECTRONIC MONITORING

My own experience with electronic monitoring of patient compliance in drug development began shortly after the commercialization of the first electronic monitor. I was thus what market theorists call an 'early adopter'. This proved to be a fortunate step, because one of the first trials in which we included use of the electronic monitor was early in the development of amlodipine, when it was still very new, with little clinical experience. A prominent academic specialist in Switzerland had organized and run a trial of amlodipine for a few weeks in patients with uncomplicated hypertension. To our surprise, he informed us that the drug was altogether without efficacy, which fact he intended to report at an upcoming international meeting. At that point, the analysis of his trial was still incomplete, so we turned to the compliance data to see if there had been especially poor compliance that might explain the lack of effectiveness.

Our most important finding from the recorded dosing histories was that the period of drug administration had ended about 2 weeks before the time when the definitive, end-of-study blood pressure measurements were made! Thus, the purported ineffectiveness of amlodipine was only a reflection of a scheduling error that might have gone undetected but for the time-stamped dosing histories of each of the patients participating in the trial. Needless to say, this information aborted the investigator's plan to announce to the world that amlodipine lacked efficacy. Had we not found this crucial error, his report would have created a considerable crisis in confidence in the new agent, which, as subsequent events have shown, has become one of the leading agents for the treatment of hypertension or angina pectoris.

My initial experience with electronic monitoring data turned out very positively, though quite differently than I had expected. It was most gratifying to be able to have the objective record of patients' dosing histories with which to resolve an awkward situation. This story emphasizes an important, but often overlooked, value of an electronically compiled dosing history: it is a primary source documentation of patients' progress through the steps specified by the trial protocol. The key factor is that the electronic monitors time-stamp every event, in a form that cannot be changed after the fact.

FIRST USE OF THE 'FORGIVING DRUG' CONCEPT

After this rather harrowing episode, the next step in the development of amlodipine came a few months later, when we began to realize that the once-a-day aspect of the amlodipine dosing regimen was hardly unique whereas its long duration of action was a unique attribute that could support a new type of claim, namely that amlodipine could maintain its therapeutic action in the face of the most common errors in compliance. We developed the data to support the view that, because the most common errors are to omit a single dose or two consecutive daily doses, amlodipine could be expected to maintain its action despite missing even two consecutive doses.

To develop support for this attribute, we undertook a very simple study with Swiss general practitioners, using the electronic monitors with their patients' various once-daily antihypertensive medications. The study was designed to show how often patients skipped one or two once-daily doses in the course of routine medical management of uncomplicated hypertension. At about the same time, a number of investigators in various parts of the world began to study the question of how long amlodipine action would continue when dosing was suddenly interrupted after some weeks of correct dosing. Meredith and Elliott in Glasgow[3], Hernandez-Hernandez et al. in Venezuela[4], and Leenen et al. in Canada[5] performed variants on a basic study design in which, after some weeks of antihypertensive treatment, placebo tablets were substituted for active drug—amlodipine or a competing agent. Importantly, these substitutions were made in a controlled and properly blinded fashion, so they have the unique rigor for inference of causality that can only be provided by randomized assignment of treatment and proper blinding. A further study on this point is expected from Kruse *et al.* in Germany. These studies showed that the post-dose duration of amlodipine action was in the vicinity of 72 hours, thus providing a generous margin for errors of omission in remedication. In contrast, none of the competing agents, which included enalapril, felodipine, and nifedipine-GITS, could maintain action for as long as 48 hours after a last-taken dose, which means that they could not forgive omission of a single dose.

The property of forgiveness for the most common errors in compliance, together with the safety profile of amlodipine, have probably played a key role in its superior performance in a variety of comparative outcome studies: amlodipine is simply far less prone to lapses in drug action than any of the presently available once-daily calcium antagonists. It is well to recall, in this context, that the original VA Cooperative Trial in hypertension, which was the first trial to show the beneficial effects of treating hypertension, was run on patients with moderate to severe hypertension who had been pre-screened to exclude grossly poor compliers and who were then treated with reserpine, which is/was the most forgiving of all antihypertensive agents with an approximately 2-week duration of action after the last-taken once-daily dose. With that extreme degree of forgiveness continuity of antihypertensive action was assured, except with the most egregious of errors, which were presumably made very unlikely by the initial screening. Thus, the commonly occurring 1–2–3 day lapses in dosing could occur with little or no impact on hypotensive action, allowing the value of blood pressure lowering to be established with statistical certainty. In contrast, clinical trials of drugs whose actions are interrupted by 1–2–3 day lapses in dosing will tend to show smaller average reductions in blood pressure and greater variance, both of which conspire to undermine statistical power.

From the research perspective, the role of superior forgiveness is clear, and gaining support. From the marketing perspective, forgiveness is a new concept that has not yet received much attention in the larger pharmaceutical market or the highest-impact journals. Yet, with the growing number of studies attesting to the long post-dose duration of action of amlodipine and the number of single-day and two-day lapses in dosing, the evidence is converging in a way that will surely kindle growing recognition of the forgiveness concept in the world of cardiovascular medicine.

THE DRUG HOLIDAY

In many ways a companion concept to forgiveness is recognition of the drug holiday as a hitherto unrecognized source of adverse events. A watershed event was the symposium on the drug holiday as a source of toxicity and adverse events, in Basel in March 1996. A valuable monograph contains the papers of the meeting plus some additional information that can be taken as the definitive establishment of the drug holiday as a factor to be reckoned with in safety evaluation of all new drugs[6].

The consequences of drug holidays vary from one drug to another. All drugs lose activity when dosing halts for more than anything from a few hours to a few days. So, with all drugs we can expect to see therapeutic action wane and disappear, sooner with some drugs, later with others. Some drugs, however, develop rebound effects when drug intake halts suddenly—e.g. central alpha blockers such as clonidine, and non-ISA beta-blockers such as propranolol or atenolol. Many drugs (e.g. the calcium antagonists) appear not to be susceptible to rebound effects although some (e.g. nifedipine) may require careful uptitration at the start of treatment to avoid overdose toxicity when the full therapeutic dose is begun suddenly; that uptitration process should probably be repeated when a drug holiday has continued for a certain time, but for how long we do not presently know. It is tempting to think, however, that many episodes of reflex tachycardia in patients taking nifedipine arise because the patient allows dosing to lapse for several days and then goes back to the usual therapeutic dose, which, after a few days without treatment, may have too potent a hypotensive action and trigger reflex adaptations. In the absence of an objective record of dosing, drug holidays usually escape clinical detection, and so the clinical events are not usually related to variations in drug intake.

A major development occurred in late 1996, when Vanhove *et al.* reported the development of drug-resistant HIV in association with the occurrences of drug holidays with one of the HIV protease inhibitors[7]. This short publication has probably had more impact per word than any other publication on the recognition of patient non-compliance as a problem to be taken seriously. In a sense it is not surprising, and indeed it was predicted a few years before[8] that drug holidays could provide the occasion for the most resistant strains of infecting microorganisms to displace the least resistant strains. In parallel with these views, the success story of directly observed therapy for tuberculosis treatment[9] is another illustration of the need for continuity in the treatment of infectious diseases.

IMPACT ON DRUG LABELING

An important development in the past several years has been the adoption of new labeling for the combined estrogen–progestagen oral contraceptives, focusing on the limits of dose timing consistent with full contraceptive efficacy and the steps patients should take when they realize that they have allowed their dosing to lapse beyond safe limits. The labeling changes differ somewhat between the UK and the USA, but the gist of the message is that a delay which exceeds 12–24 hours (12 in the UK, 24 in the USA) is an indication for the patient to institute use of backup barrier contraception (condom and/or diaphragm) for the next 7 days, while resuming dosing as soon as the lapse is identified. Patients are informed, when they have missed one or two doses, to take one missed dose together with the next scheduled dose, and use backup barrier methods for the next 7 days. If they have missed more than two doses, they are instructed to discard the pill pack, use backup barrier methods until their next period commences, and then start a new pack[10].

The important point in all this is not the details *per se* but that there is a body of experimental evidence, based on controlled substitution of placebo pills for active pills, on how long the steroidal blockade of ovulation persists, and that this evidence forms the basis for the label recommendations for 'how much compliance is enough?' and 'what should I do when my compliance has not been good enough?'. These labeling changes and the type of studies on which they are based are an important milestone in the path toward full-disclosure, user-friendly labeling.

It is of course noteworthy that the combined oral contraceptives are the pharmaceuticals with the greatest cumulative use, and products where the impact of poor compliance is readily grasped by essentially everyone without need for professional-level education. Clearly, we need to take this lesson and apply it to other chronic-use prescription pharmaceuticals, so that both patients and caregivers are as informed as the underlying scientific data permit about the limits of compliance consistent with full benefits, and what to do when those limits have been exceeded. Such information can allow patients who deviate substantially from the recommended regimen to return to correct dosing with the least perturbation and risk.

LOOKING AHEAD

The data from electronic monitoring have revealed several pragmatically important aspects of pharmaceutical care. As with other advances in medicine, sound methods are essential for progress, even if the conclusions drawn from the new information are not entirely welcome—i.e. that there is so much poor and partial compliance. This new information has, however, taught us that we need to look beyond the compliance numbers to understand their clinical impact, and to focus on those errors that have the potential to change outcomes of treatment. As these new views are assimilated, we can expect emphasis to shift away from reflex repetition of the presumed but ill-documented advantages of once-daily dosing and to move toward the more realistic perspective created by the concept of forgiveness. The aim, after all, is not to achieve perfection in compliance but to achieve the full benefits of rationally prescribed prescription drugs. Part of that goal can be achieved by prescribing more forgiving pharmaceuticals, and part will have to depend on the success of efforts to improve compliance. There is evidence that feedback of objective measurement data to patients can help them to improve compliance[11]. It opens a new vista, hopefully not a false one, that previously disappointing efforts to improve compliance[12,13] can be overcome by using objective data on daily dosing times as a way to link dosing to routines in the daily lives of the patients.

We should not have unrealistic expectations that a panacea awaits those who start to use electronic monitoring data in programs of compliance management. Nevertheless, the combined use of more forgiving pharmaceuticals and data-driven patient management should bring the greatest number of patients under the umbrella of effective medical treatment. Parallel effort should go into development of ultra-long-acting medicines, a good example of which is the silicone rubber implant for progestin-only contraception, which transformed progestin-only contraception from the least forgiving (in its oral form) to the most forgiving (in its implant form) pharmaceutical, with correspondingly large improvements in its contraceptive effectiveness, transforming it from the least to the most effective steroidal contraceptive[14].

Will effective medication management/counseling compete with forgiving drugs? In a narrow sense each represents a path toward the same goal— correct usage of prescription drugs—so in that sense they are competitive, but today the main problem is not 'which approach should we choose?' but lack of appreciation of the prevalence of poor compliance and the problems it creates. Thus, the big hurdle is not to fashion the technologically best solution to the problem but to stimulate awareness that the problem exists. With that as the focus, the development of potentially competing approaches has the potential to promote awareness of the problem of achieving effective usage of prescription pharmaceuticals.

REFERENCES

1. Efron B. Foreword to the Limburg Compliance Symposium. *Stat Med* **17**: 249–50, 1998.
2. Lasagna L, Hutt PB. Health care, research, and regulatory impact of non-compliance. In: *Compliance in Medical Practice and Clinical Trials*. Eds: Cramer JA, Spilker B. New York: Raven Press, 1991, pp. 393–403.
3. Meredith PA, Elliott HL. Therapeutic coverage: reducing the risks of partial compliance. *Br J Clin Pract* **May** (Suppl 73): 13–17, 1994.
4. Hernandez-Hernandez R, Armas de Hernandez MJ, Armas-Padilla MC, Carvajal AR, Guerrero-Pajuelo J. The effects of missing a dose of enalapril versus amlodipine on ambulatory blood pressure. *Blood Press Monitor* **1**: 1121–6, 1996.
5. Leenen FHH, Fourney A, Notman G, Tanner J. Persistence of anti-hypertensive effect after 'missed doses' of calcium antagonist with long (amlodipine) vs short (diltiazem) elimination half-life. *Br J Clin Pharmacol* **41**: 83–8, 1996.

6. Meyer UA, Peck CC (eds). *The Drug Holiday Pattern of Noncompliance in Clinical Trials: Challenge to Conventional Concepts of Drug Safety and Efficacy.* Washington DC: Center for Drug Development Science, Georgetown University, 1997.
7. Vanhove GF, Schapiro JM, Winters MA, Merigan TC, Blaschke TF. Patient compliance and drug failure in protease inhibitor monotherapy. *JAMA* **276**: 1955–6, 1996.
8. Urquhart J. Variable patient compliance in ambulatory trials—nuisance, threat, opportunity. *J Antimicrob Chemother* **32**: 643–9, 1993.
9. Weis SE, Slocum PC, Blais FX, King B, Nunn M, Matney GB, Gomez E, Foresman BH. The effect of directly observed therapy on the rates of drug resistance and relapse in tuberculosis. *N Engl J Med* **330**: 1179–84, 1994.
10. Guillebaud J. Any questions? *BMJ* **307**: 617, 1993.
11. Schneider M-P, Burnier M. Un suivi quotidien de l'observance therapeutique est-il possible a domicile? Resultats d'une etude pilote. *Schweiz Med Wochenschr* **127** (suppl 88): 122, 1997.
12. Sackett DL, Haynes RB, Gibson ES, Taylor DW, Roberts RS, Johnson AL, Hackett BC, Turford C, Mossey J. Randomized trials of compliance-improving strategies in hypertension. In *Patient Compliance.* Ed. Lasagna L. Mount Kisco (NY): Futura, 1976, pp. 1–19.
13. Haynes RB, McKibbon KA, Kanani R. Systematic review of randomised trials of interventions to assist patients to follow prescriptions for medications. *Lancet* **348**: 383–6, 1996.
14. Urquhart J. Can delivery systems deliver value in the new pharmaceutical marketplace? *Br J Clin Pharmacol* **44**: 413–19, 1997.

Index

Note: page numbers in *italics* refer to figures and tables

Index compiled by Jill C. Halliday